Remedy

Title: **Remedy**

Author: **Norah al-Sbeiy**

Category: **Public Health**

Publisher: **Madarek Publishing House**

First edition: May, 2024

ISBN: 978 - 614 - 429 - 543 - 4

Translated by: Hala Ali

تمت ترجمة هذا الكتاب ضمن

مبادرة ترجم

Tarjim Initiative

Madarek

Madarek Publishing House

مدارك

دار مدارك للنشر

8470 Othman Bin Affan St, Al Taawun Dist, Riyadh, Saudi Arabia

Zip Code: 3844 - 12478 Riyadh, Saudi Arabia Tel: +966 114541148

mdrek.com read@mdrek.com DarMadarek

Remedy

Norah al-Sbeiy

Translated by: Hala Ali

Contents

Dedication

To my father, who came to me one day with an intramuscular injection and said, "Why should I go to clinics when I have a nurse at home?"

To my mother, who greets me every day by saying, "Welcome our nurse."

To everyone whose question remained unanswered when they said: "I would like to ask you about nursing. I got accepted into the nursing school, and I am afraid."

Introduction

When we consider our trajectories and the choices we make every day, we realise that life is nothing but a constant stream of decisions and experiences. However, we must also acknowledge that not all of these decisions were chosen by us! While we have the power to make some choices, others are beyond our control.

Nursing chose me, and I studied it for five years, two of which I spent trying to escape from it. Until I met patients, experienced several lives within my life, and lived feelings beyond my own. After that, I learned what nursing and remediation are all about, as they not only mean providing medicine or food but also giving care and attention; some patients only need someone to talk to, and this is what I did. Now is the time to break my silence and do more than listen. I will convey to you what I experienced in the course of my study and inside hospitals.

It is one thing to pass through experiences but quite another to go through them! If you pass through experiences, you are standing still in one place, and your situation is unaltered. It means having encounters and watching moments pass before your eyes without the slightest movement from you until you decide to straighten your back, strengthen your feet, and strive to live those experiences. Only then will you learn something unique from each one of them and treasure it. So, you peacefully let go of all things in peace, while what you learned remains untouched and resistant and excels in giving you a different meaning to your life, planting roses in wounds and creating hope out of pain!

Being a writer for the first time, I faced many obstacles and fears about publishing this book. I remember meeting a doctor who laughed as he told me that he had spent more than ten years working in medicine and had not thought of writing a single book, so how would an inexperienced nurse like me write one?! I was discouraged then, as if all I needed were words like these to make the anxiety I felt build up inside me and stop my pursuit.

Yet, every time I imagined how one of my lines would affect

a nursing student, a junior nurse, or even someone outside the nursing profession,

I go back to my desk, sit in front of my laptop, and continue what I started. I believe neither white hair nor wrinkles qualify an individual to write a book. Rather, all experiences are worthy of being published. Perhaps they will inspire one person or motivate another, and this is all I hope for.

In this humble book are stories of situations I experienced, in addition to findings I reached after a thorough meditation following each situation. This meditation includes a psychological study, research I had read, or even an opinion I had expressed.

It is unnecessary- dear reader- that you work in the health sector to read this book, as its language is simple, and its medical terminology is explained in the margins of each page.

Notice:

On one of my training days, while I was preparing the operating room table, the patient asked me before anesthesia: "Are you Saudi?" I replied: "Yes." She smiled in astonishment, then said that it was the first time that she had noticed the presence of an entirely Saudi medical staff!

The magnitude of this pleasant yet strange incident inspired some of the topics of this book, which will include letters of thanks and gratitude addressed to the Arab healthcare givers with whom I dealt In recognition of their services and an indication of their high-quality work, which may be hidden from many.

And if you are not interested in that -dear reader- of course, you can always turn the page and move on to the next topic.

Norah, the Pediatrician!

As a child, I used the floor as a bed for dolls. I would look after them as if I were in a medical nursery, moving between one doll and the other, examining one of them, and giving medicine to the other while brushing their heads. I only stopped when I thought that the few minutes of my work had run out, and now was the time to return to reality. I repeated this show daily until my mother predicted my tendency to go into the medical profession. Since then, and until I graduated from high school, my mother started calling me: "Noura, the pediatrician!" And when someone asked me about my ambitions after high school, I answered hastily: "I will study medicine- *Inshallah*." Indeed, I applied for the Faculty of Medicine at every university in the Kingdom. I was determined to study only this specialization, and if I got rejected, I should not go further with my studies! Until it was time to apply to our local university, and of course,

I chose medicine as my first choice and sole desire. Then, after my family convinced me, I added two other majors as a backup plan through which I could be involved with the medical major: Nursing School- as a second choice- and Business Management- as a third choice. As was the case, I got accepted into business management and nursing. However, I was waiting for my name to move on to a higher level to get accepted into the college I chose first, but it did not happen.

School days came bearing a heavy burden, as there is no burden in the world equal to the burden of pursuing something unwanted. Three days later, the process of what I call manual transfer began[(1)]. I resolved to submit my papers to be transferred to the Faculty of Medicine, and I was handed the transfer form and was about to fill it out and hand it in immediately, but a subtle feeling told me: Slow down!

I grabbed the form and started thinking about nursing and comparing it to medicine.

---

(1) Submitting a request to transfer to another college by manually handing over the papers after making available a certain number of seats in each major.

I had a strange feeling: How did I think I was designed for one thing and went on thinking solely about it, never letting my mind think about anything else? It was as if I lived in a locked box with no source of light except for a small lamp that I clung to, and I spent great effort and time to preserve it, then discovered that life outside this box was vast and more capacious where the light filled the place, and was not limited to that lamp.

As I was weighing this on my mind, I met a colleague and a friend of mine studying medicine, and I was happy to tell them what was occupying my mind, hoping they would help me overcome my hesitation. One of them said: "Choose medicine, of course." I replied with a question: "And what about nursing?" She replied with excitement: "Are you serious, Norah!? A nurse is a maid in the hospital.[1]" I was extremely surprised that I laughed at the time, but deep inside, I felt a biting cold despite the bright sun out there.

I thought that people's views towards nursing had evolved a lot from what they used to be, but these lingering ideas surprised

(1) I dedicate my greetings to this colleague with all my love and respect, hoping that my words will not be understood as resentment towards her.

me and made me think: How can such ideas and terminology be steadfast until now? Yes, these terms were circulated previously when the health sector was limited to the doctor and the nurse, and nursing had no other role than carrying out the doctor's orders only, and this contributed - in my opinion - to looking at nursing as a secondary major or a service work. However, the diversity of multiple health specialties showed the importance of each specialty on its own, as all of them are vital and strive to serve the patient.

I started studying nursing, and this question still occupied my mind: Why do some negative ideas about nursing persist until now? Until I attended a course whose introduction discussed the history of nursing in the West.

The dark ages of nursing[1]! That was one of the main headlines that grabbed my attention.

That was the dark period of nursing between the years 1500 AD- 1860 AD, in which nursing lived its lowest and darkest

---

(1) Claros, Edith, Kimberly Foisy, and Teresa Deam Nursing History and Theory. Jones and Bartlett, 2013, Pp. 59.

times, when the religious schools that were responsible at that time for teaching the nursing profession stopped teaching it[1], and no longer could anyone be trained to have the necessary knowledge for the practice of nursing healthcare. Hospitals, therefore, resorted to other ways through which they attracted workers, even if they were untrained.

Indeed, the first of those were of the illiterate class, and despite that, they were few in number; they were able to stigmatize nursing as a harsh, rude, and reckless profession because of the way they treated patients.

Within a few days, several individuals, most of whom were immoral and alcoholics, poured into the hospitals. As an American journalist, Phil Donau described it as follows: "When a woman could not be a gambler, a prostitute, or a thief, she would often become a nurse." In an attempt to meet the needs of hospitals, the law has made healthcare one of the options of

(1) Nursing began in the Western world as it did in the Islamic world, from a religious perspective, as the nursing movement began with teaching nuns simple nursing skills in religious schools, after which they were allowed to provide care on a limited scale.

community services for criminals to choose instead of going to prison. So, tell me: How do you imagine those who worked in this profession at the time?

Despite this information, I never found an answer to my question, and I only believed that it was the arbitrariness of the beginnings. During my research, I found a turning point in that dark age, with which a man immortalized this image deeply: Charles Dickens, the author of the famous series of stories at the time titled *Martin Chuzzlewit.*

Dickens›s works had a huge readership for the simplicity they were famous for and their intriguing style of description of reality. Of course, a writer of his fame would not miss the opportunity to write about that foul situation.

He became interested in observing one of the nurses look after patients at his friend's house. Despite being illiterate, alcoholic, rude, and sometimes a thief, he was intrigued by her work. The nurse in the story is named Sairey Gamp, and the author vividly describes her unattractive appearance and cruel behavior. Unfortunately, the character was later portrayed in a children's animation series, which promoted a negative image of the nursing profession.

Media power! This is the answer I have been looking for to my question: Why do some negative ideas about nursing still exist today? In the early twentieth century, electronic mass media models were dubbed "The hypodermic needle" or "The magic bullet" theories, which portrayed media messages as strong drugs or lethal weapons that would have profound effects on a helpless audience. They have a strong influence on the minds of the audience, who completely take hold of the information as a fact. In an article titled "Cultural Indicators: Violence Profile,(1)" I found some of the actual effects of the media based on psychological and social studies. The most important of these effects are:

- The priming effect: It suggests that the messages of the mass media stimulate the recall of previously stored ideas, knowledge, opinions, or experiences associated in some way with the content of the message. It works like a primer, which, despite

(1) Gerbner, G., Gross, L., Jackson-Beeck, M., Jeffries-Fox, S., & Signorielli, N. (1978). Cultural indicators: Violence profile, no. 9. Journal of Communication, 28, 176–207.

its small size, can trigger many ideas stored within our memories over the years.

- Agenda-setting (laying the grounds): This theory suggests that the media does not affect what people believe in, but rather what they think, by choosing and reinforcing what issues are given the most attention. In other words, your beliefs may be sound but you may, like other people, you may have different conventions, whether good or bad, and these networks work to reinforce your conventions and position them among your beliefs until they shape your beliefs and opinions.

- The Cultivation hypothesis (instilling ideas): It suggests that over time, heavy exposure to television may result in perceiving the version of reality depicted on television as a reflection of the real world. The intense crowding of the mass media cultivates this belief. So, the audience starts behaving according to what they see and believes that the course of real life is identical to what is displayed on TV. For example, we may be biased against a certain group of people because we are accustomed to a bad image presented about people similar to them on the screen, so we unconsciously believe that it is their reality!

To Conclude, the effects of the media are more powerful than we think, and the messages it injects are more dangerous than we realize. So, what if they inject messages related to the health specialties responsible for our health?

Unfortunately, the image of nursing was not the only message that was misrepresented and implanted in many people's minds. Medical misconceptions are also represented in a lot of stories and scenes. There is, for instance, the use of electroconvulsive therapy for mental health problems and portraying it to us as a terrifying torture scene.

And when I attended one of these sessions, I stood at a long distance for fear of the patient's agitation. However, this session has a preparation similar to the preparation for any surgery. There is an anesthesia staff, a nursing staff, and an attending physician, as the patient is under general anesthesia. After that, the doctor sticks two pieces of conductive material to pass a mild electric current through the brain; the patient wakes up immediately.

In addition to other misconceptions that I noticed, such as the use of resuscitation equipment, the method of cardiopulmonary resuscitator for each age group, and others which many rely on as a source of their information.

Media messages are so effective and powerful that they reach faster than the correct information, as was the case with the character of "Sairey Gamp," who resembled a bad image that led to disrespecting this profession. And even though we have an honorable Islamic history of nursing that began with the venerable companion Rufayda Al-Aslamia who was honored and admired by the Messenger- may God bless him and grant him peace- after he ordered to pitch a tent for her to look after the wounded inside it, this history was not documented by the media, and therefore, was not rooted in the mind of the public.

What I ask of you, dear reader, and what I would like all of us to be reminded of, is to review our postulates and ideas before making any judgment. We may be victims of the influence of the media, so we unconsciously adopt ideas which would affect our view of the world around us. If you are wondering what happened later with the decision I left pending, I handed back the transfer form to the manager and moved on, attempting to find myself within the corridors of Nursing College. I am still discovering myself in this world. So, I did not become Noura, the pediatrician? Rather, I became a nurse and granddaughter of Rufayda Al-Aslamia.

The Ozone Hole[1]

Have you ever wondered: How does change happen? How could an idea on the verge of falling apart rise to reality?

In an English language class with a cold atmosphere and strong lighting, which a non-Arab teacher gave to many students of different cultures, one of them asked a question that was sufficient to clarify one of the paradoxes between one culture and another and between people's interests and future aspirations. She asked the teacher: "How many children do you have?" The teacher's response was unexpected and left everyone shocked.

(1) Ozone hole is a region of marked thinning of the ozone layer in the Earth's atmosphere. This phenomenon chiefly occurs in Antarctica, attributed to the chemical action of chlorofluorocarbons and other atmospheric pollutants. The hole, however, does not mean the absence of the layer, that is, it is not a hole as the name indicates, but rather the process of draining this layer as a result of chemical reactions. Studies have shown that there is a direct relationship between population density and the expansion of this hole.

She frowned as if trying to squeeze her forehead to extract some answer buried there and eventually responded disapprovingly: "How can I have a child when the population density on Earth is increasing? And with its increase, the ozone hole is expanding."

She continued to talk about the great significance of this decision on public health and that she could not bear the consequences of her decision to have a single child coming out of her womb when all of us are under the threat of being aborted from the womb of this planet. She finished her justification amid our astonishment that slipped through our eyes and mouths. A group of us laughed, while another doubted their comprehension due to the difference in language, and a group- to which I belonged- was frightened by the idea. I was not panicked at the idea so much as at the depth of conviction it instilled.

We may fear expressing our ideas that are contradictory to the norm. We may doubt ourselves at the first condemnation we read in the faces of the crowd, declaring the abandonment of those ideas to a region of stagnation, forgetting that the greatest inventions and ideas began with people who spent a large part of their lives amid accusations and judgments, who dragged themselves out of it with on-going persistence and determination. So, how does change happen?

It is said that the only constant in life is change. Yes! We live a change every day, be it slight or profound, and those changes are deeply rooted in our lives and constantly change them. We have always managed to rise amid a new change that we neither remember nor recognize how it happened. So, allow me, dear reader, to tell you of these secret beginnings, as I always believe.

Change happens when people believe in an idea to the point of obsession; they dedicate their lives to it through innovation and creativity in the quest for bridges capable of conveying their interest to those around them.

Many scientists and innovators lived on the verge of madness to prove their creativity to the world, and the physician Werner Forsmann is a great example of that. He invented cardiac catheterization decades ago. When he suggested this idea, he was accused of madness, which prompted him to prove what was in his mind in every way possible. Do you know how he proved to his colleagues and the whole world the effectiveness of this idea?

He carried on an experiment on himself! Yes, he risked his life and inserted a medical tube starting from the artery of his hand and reaching the chambers of the right side of his heart. He was subsequently awarded the Nobel Peace Prize in Medicine. Certainly, our use of cardiac catheterization in hospitals these days is clear evidence of the success of his invention, which emerged to the world in 1929 AD.

And here is Professor Mark Ferguson, who discovered a substance that helps heal wounds; and when one of the institutions agreed to fund his discovery, provided that it was proven, he did not hesitate to wound both hands and put his material on one of them while leaving the other so that the wound covered with that material healed faster and proved his discovery.

Do we still resist change because we are in fear of it?

The writer Tony Buzan, in his book *Embracing change*, suggested an interesting equation:

experience + event + evaluation + study + application = success

The experience of applying one of the ideas that possess our minds is the first degree of the equation of success and change. Moreover, this experience will inevitably generate an event that needs evaluation and analysis, and there is no problem in seeking help from the people we trust. After reviewing these assessments, we can apply the idea with higher quality once, twice, or ten times until perfection... This is how the world is convinced of an idea so that change and success can happen.

Moreover, there is another equation that I am very familiar with:

Vision + skills + motivation + appropriate resources + work plan = change

Each side of this equation is important in bringing about successful change. If the clear vision is dropped, it results in confusion; if skills are dropped, anxiety is the outcome; if motivation is dropped, resistance results; if the sources are dropped, discouragement and nullification are the outcome; and if the action plan fell through, the beginning is mostly wrong. Finally, if we choose to drop this entire equation without starting it, others will inevitably apply it and bring about a change they chose. As with the ozone hole. If we choose to have children, this teacher will abstain from doing it to prove something that will inevitably bring change.

Dear Nurse Sarah,

A Nurse in the Emergency Department

Thank you for your effort and dedication to your profession... We were used to seeing Sarah in the triage unit, and I never forget when we asked her about that; she said: «Employees cannot be placed randomly because the triage unit is a critical area on which the later management of the case is based. Rather, specific people are selected after passing several demanding tests.» It is noteworthy that Sarah was one of only three people who passed these tests in fierce competition, including many of the hospital›s nursing staff. She is now qualified to head the triage unit, where patients are divided into urgent, non-urgent, or even emergent cases.

A Tourist Attraction in Our College!

Suppose I told you to ask anyone on the streets about the most memorable spots in Egypt, France, or China, for example. In that case, they will respond with knit eyebrows and an exclamation denoting surprise: Of course, The Pyramids, the Eiffel Tower, and the Great Wall of China! But, if I superseded the question and the person asked with one of our college students- Applied Medical Sciences College– and asked her about the teacher who is embraced by the college, she would immediately answer: Go to Dr. Ola's office! So, dear readers, allow me to take you on a tour of this famous landmark.

The archipelago of our college is mainly distinguished by its strategic location as its northern wall adjoins another office, and from the south, it overlooks the beautiful view of the façade of the university health clinic. At the same time, from the southwest, there is a small room considered a mine for means and files, and finally, on the northwest side, there is a narrow window in which a glorious printer is located!

This landmark is considered a historical archive of all the times the college has gone through and a warm home when the strong winds of tests storm.

I have always thought about Dr. Ola's splendid conduct with us, and about her unlimited trust in us, to the extent that her office became our favorite spot whether to outline a certain project, ask for help in other courses, or even rid ourselves of the thoughts that occupy our minds. Some may consider that what the doctor provides us does not really count. Still, I believe that providing moral support is a great and profound idea, especially if it extends over a long time and if this simple support remains steadfast and unchanged, no matter how circumstances change. As I remember this kindness, another example of support and giving comes into my mind: the knight behind it, Dr. Sayyed, who came temporarily for a few days to lecture us on Census when the assigned course teacher excused himself. As soon as he noticed our dread of the Census course, which coincided with our bad marks in it, he decided to voluntarily devote additional time to summarize the entire course down to what did not exceed the space of the whiteboard centered in the classroom. Not only that, but he also suggested conducting a test that included the basics of the Census to raise our grades in it.

I recall the moment when he stood for an hour after that test holding in his hand the stack of papers that did not receive a full mark, and he called out the names of the girls (who did not receive a perfect score) one by one, with his euphonious voice amidst the prevailing silence. Our limbs trembled. We did not expect this kind of embarrassment. However, within a few moments, this embarrassment became a feeling of appreciation and gratitude. He did not call on us to scold us, give us a sharp look, teach us a lesson, or make an example of us. Instead, he meant to clarify to each of us individually the mistakes that led her to lose marks.

I still remember my particular feelings when it was my turn. At that time, I commenced indicating my mistake and explaining the right approach and the correct answer. He, then, said to me: "Well, so you are certainly aware of the right approach?" "Yes," I replied. So, he crossed out the previous mark with a red pen and replaced it with a full mark! Because as long as the student understands the right approach and the correct answer, nothing else matters. By the way, I returned to his summaries four years later while preparing for the Professional Classification Exam for nursing!

Many names jammed in my memory and had me spend a long time reflecting on the great benefit that such support and giving can yield, even in the simplest matters. Then, I remembered one of Stephen Covey's famous principles mentioned in his book, *The Seven Habits of Highly Effective People*[(1)], which is the fourth habit: thinking about mutual benefit, which includes the following intellectual perspectives of human interaction:

- Win/ Win
- Win /Lose
- Lose/Win
- Lose/Lose
- Win /Win or no deal

(1) Covey, Stephen R, The Seven Habits of Highly Effective People: Restoring the Character Ethic. New York, Simon and Schuster, 1989, Pp. 231.

This means that any interaction between individuals or groups does not take place far from one of the previous ideational perspectives, and the individual may draw plans to follow one of them before initiating any interaction or communication, or it could take place spontaneously in a certain track. For example, when an individual meets a colleague at school or work, they may chart out a tendency for their relationship to be competitive with a (win/lose) end. If they win, a colleague should lose, or they may choose the opposite perspective by winning their colleague's affection.

If we wonder where the positions of giving that I detailed earlier lie, we will find them in the win/ win perspective. This perspective is all about the methods, decisions, or even personal initiatives used to achieve satisfaction or benefit both parties. The win/win perspective requires a combination of wisdom, a balanced heart, and a courageous and considerate personality.

How many times have you had a professor who turns lectures into personal battles, using them to boast about themselves and belittle their students? They constantly remind us that they are at higher levels, consequently making us feel disconnected from them and their courses. So, why should we expend effort and time owning something everyone can achieve, as long as there is room for others to win? I am not saying that fair competition should be eliminated, as every reality and objective has a unique perspective. Rather, I am referring to the marginalization of the win principle and considering it a kind of loss.

On the contrary, it is considered one of the foundations of collective leadership and collaborative learning to achieve success- by God's will. Therefore, had it not been for the generous giving of faculty members, they would not be able to witness our success and feel proud of it. They earned our success, and we earned their generosity, and vice versa.

Dear Dr. Jalal,

A Family Physician in the Emergency Department

Thank you! Because when you are with the patient, you dedicate most of your time and effort to health education.

I remember that patient who was suffering from back pain; I thought she came out with a long list of medications and ointments after about 40 minutes in the clinic, but in fact, he did not prescribe anything to her except some tips for physical activity that should help her to maintain a healthy body. He spent all those long minutes solely in health education because he had always believed it was as important as medicine.

HESI

It seems that we are constantly moving in gridlock, rushing through our days amid the clangor of tasks and the flashing lights of plans. Our minds, lives, and paths are all cluttered with monuments of ideas, varying in height depending on how much effort we put into bringing them to life.

We were the first building block in one of the emerging edifices in our college, in the establishment of which we had to go through many challenges. One of these challenges was the HESI[1] test, which was one of the requirements of the nursing program in our college that is conjoint with the College of Nursing at the University of Massachusetts in the United States of America. HESI

(1)8 Health Education Systems Incorporated is a United States company that provides exams and other study material to help prepare student nurses for their professional licensure exam. Schools often use HESI to help predict the student's likelihood of success in tests such as the NCLEX-RN.

is a computerized test operated over the internet. It measures the extent of our understanding of medical information and its application within several situations limited to texts that do not exceed one or two lines. It is pretty similar to the NCLEX test and the Saudi Nursing Licensing Exam (SNLE).

I still remember in detail the long duration of each test and how we sat firmly before the computer screen while the sound of clicks filled the place, as our fingers moved between the keyboard at times and the mouse at others, and sometimes on the surface of the table, as an attempt to release our tension. Our beginnings were disappointing. We prepared for the first test in many ways, but the result was the same. "I apologize for disturbing you, but we just received an email with your marks for the first three tests of this semester, and your success rate in all of them was lower than the expected or even required level!" said the head of the department with great astonishment, and what made that astonishment even more disappointing was the loudness of our laughter after she finished. Yes... We knew that we did not perform well on our tests, but we did not exactly expect those results, so we had no better reaction than to laugh.

The next semester began, and the clamor of our laughter turned into a grim amount of stress and random work to figure out the best way to pass this test. Multiple sources, summaries, and the heap of questions filling the desktops were all the details shared by more than fifty students who wanted only to pass that test. We tried our best to cancel the test and suggested this through multiple letters and emails to the college dean. However, the head of the department had a different perspective and rejected our suggestion. In fact, he even doubled the test percentage from 15% to 30% of our total mark, justifying it by saying that we needed nothing more than motivation. By doubling the percentage, the challenge doubled, motivating us to put more effort until we succeeded.

This has provoked our indignation and resentment because we were not expecting an incentive veiled as a challenge. Rather, we were waiting for the test to be cancelled. Yet, our agitation resulted in nothing. We grew more anxious as days passed, but we had to curb that stress and make more progress in our preparation for the test.

During those days, two of the teaching staff in the faculty

chose to motivate us, but in different ways. The first one sent an audio recording of her young child praying for us, overflowing with innocence and kindness. The second postponed her encouragement until the night of the test by sending us a letter to motivate us, in which she expressed her confidence in our competence and hard work. They utilized various techniques, such as encouraging us with challenges, love, hope, a sense of responsibility, and trust, all with the same goal in mind - to instill confidence in us so that we could pass the test with satisfactory results.

But wait...! Do you think this was just the end? And that we were satisfied with those results alone?

While we were still in the middle of the stressful exams, emails continued reaching us uninterrupted, and mobile screens kept vibrating nonstop. Many calls were coming in, all for the same end: the administrative staff at the University of Massachusetts were astonished and wanted to verify our actual marks. What is happening? Why this panic and desire for certainty? Shall I tell you what happened?

Our average marks in the Maternal and Child Health Nursing course exceeded the average marks of male and female students in America by three hundred grades. That is, we, who were experiencing this test for the first time, were ahead by three hundred points of those who preceded us in such tests. Not only that, but we also were ahead of them in our penultimate test by more than seven hundred points. Their average marks in the Community Health course were 919, and ours were 1649 points! We were over the moon, and we started wondering whether this was real or not.

This success remained behind closed doors at the college and did not appear publicly. Yet, we proudly showed it at a different time and place after we took the examination of the Saudi Commission for Health Specialties. During my internship year, only thirteen female students from our batch applied. As you may know, preparing for this exam is one of the toughest periods that any medical student goes through. We must revisit everything we learned in all major specialties and use various strategies to study them. Neither one nor two days, or even two weeks, are sufficient for this. It took me two months to prepare for the exam, and some of my friends took even longer.

However, we finally passed, praise be to God, and it was only a matter of days before it was announced that our university representatives had obtained first place with the highest average score in the Saudi Commission for Health Specialties nursing test. We were thankful that the dean of the College, the University President, and the Minister of Health himself celebrated our success, and we felt that we were finally reaping the fruits of our hard work and determination, which we sowed since we have turned the tides with the HESI test. Even now, whenever I recollect those days, the incentives given back then, which varied in strength and type, always come to my mind. We all passed the test, but what was our motivation? Is it the feeling of challenge that the dean intended to instill? Is it the love and hope that the doctor's child delivered? Or is it the sense of responsibility and trust the other doctor conveyed? Objectively and far from casting judgment on those motivators, I have always seen that responsibility and trust are stronger than the sense of competition and challenge. I think that empowering someone with confidence is more effective than challenging them because a challenge can sometimes imply doubt in their abilities. On the other hand, when you inspire someone to take on responsibility, you show that you have faith in them and their capabilities.

David McClelland, a psychologist and theorist, once posed a profound question: What truly motivates us? This question aims to reach the foundation and roots of motivation rather than circumstantial matters like having a job, a family, or a hobby. McClelland proposes three roots that he believes are the main driving motivators we all need, regardless of gender, cultural background, or age. These roots dominate us, control our minds, and unconsciously induce our actions.

The first of these motivations is related to people, which is affiliation; the second has to do with success, which is achievement; the third is about control and responsibility, and we can call it power(1).

Individuals who are motivated by affiliation have a strong desire to belong to a group and feel loved. They tend to conform to the group's norms and values and prefer collaboration over

(1) Quilliam, Susan. What Makes People Tick?: The Ultimate Guide to Personality Types. Element, 2003. Pp. 15.

competition. Therefore, they may find their group's opinion to be a motivating factor in decision-making. They are more likely to be motivated to participate in activities that require teamwork and cooperation.

Achievers, on the other hand, have a strong need to set and achieve difficult goals. They calculate the risks before they start work. In contrast to the affiliation type of people, achievers often like to work alone without a group.

The last type includes those who prefer power and influence and find their motivation controlling and influencing others. They enjoy competing and winning and prefer competitiveness more than collaboration to be distinctive and gain appreciation.

People are motivated by different things, and each of us has a unique motivator that drives us. Discovering your core motivator can save you the trouble of attempting to motivate yourself with the wrong things. If you are driven by a sense of belonging, make sure to surround yourself with your group when you feel overwhelmed by a task. If achievement motivates you, don't waste your time on small tasks when you can achieve greater things. If you seek influence and power, engage in fair competition with your peers. How about you? Take a moment to tap into your subconscious and consider what type of motivation drives you to do your best.

Dear Nurse Marwa,

A Nurse in the Mental Health Inpatient Department

I wanted to take a moment to express my gratitude for your placid and kind demeanor towards the patients in the Department of Psychological Health Inpatient. Despite the common approach of imposing medical authority driven by the e conviction that it makes it easier to handle patients, you choose to maintain a low tone of voice and speak serenely with all patients. Your approach is truly appreciated and makes a positive impact on the well-being of those in your care.

Cloak of Shame

I woke up to the sound of my alarm clock, greeted by the peacefulness of a new day. Today, I was assigned to work in the newborn nursery ward, where innocence, purity reign, and prejudice have no place.

My duties included taking care of the babies and preparing them for life. This involved tasks such as clearing their nose and mouth cavities of fluids, assessing their reflexes to ensure their nervous system was healthy, and measuring their bodies to ensure they were within normal ranges. Additionally, I was responsible for feeding and cleaning them. Despite the workload, my love for these precious little ones made every task worthwhile. Caring for them brought out our most tender and intimate sides, and it felt like we were doing it instinctively.

Our promptness never ceased until we were sternly cautioned

by a nurse in a harsh tone to not touch the child due to a possible hepatitis infection. We hastened to wash our hands out of concern for our safety. Later on, we learned that infants born to mothers with infectious diseases are placed in isolation as a precautionary health measure until it's determined whether or not they have the infection. The infant was in isolation with many red papers hanging on his small incubator, indicating that he tested positive for hepatitis B. This experience made me realize that in mental health hospitals, patients are often placed in isolation not by concrete walls but by the attitudes of the nurses, who create an insurmountable barrier that blocks their acceptance of those patients.

I also recalled the advice given by one of our clinical instructors regarding treating psychiatric patients and all patients in general. The first step is to accept them, and the key to that is understanding and accepting ourselves in the first place.

Sometimes, life throws unexpected challenges at us, and the least we deserve is to shed off the toxic shame imposed upon us by society. The hospital should always be a haven for everyone, regardless of their circumstances. Is it so difficult to accept this?

To begin, it's important to accept ourselves as we are. This means getting to know ourselves, appreciating our points of strength, and then extending that same acceptance and appreciation to others. As part of our mental health implementation, we participated in an activity called "Self-awareness," which helped us better understand ourselves and learn to accept ourselves and others.

Step 1: Create a simplified drawing of yourself.

Step 2: Use the drawing to answer the following questions.

- In the head area: Write down a talent or ability bestowed upon you by God.
- Eyebrow area using your favorite color: Draw it with the typical angle of your eyebrows.
- Right eye: briefly describe yourself using one or two words.
- Left eye: In five years from now, how would you describe yourself in just a word or two?
- Nose: Name your favorite fragrances.
- Lips: Mention your motto or life philosophy.

- Right ear: Share a compliment that you would appreciate receiving.
- Left ear: Write a story about you that you would never like to hear.
- Neck: Mention one or two barriers to building your independence.
- Right shoulder: Write down the people who feel responsible for you and the people or things you are responsible for.
- Left shoulder: list any present responsibilities that may be hindering you from discovering your true self.
- Chest area: List the names of people or things you love and feel vulnerable around.
- Right hand:
- Summarize your abilities in a few words.
- Left hand: briefly describe some of your vulnerabilities.
- Middle area: Can you briefly describe your typical eating habits?

- Pelvic area: How do you adapt to life changes?
- Thighs and legs: Can you explain what your major strength points are in life?
- Knees: Explain how you typically respond to making mistakes in life.

Feet: List the names of individuals who have helped you stay grounded and realistic.

Step 3: Consider a scenario where you have only seven days to live. Create a list of things you want to accomplish during these seven days.

Step 4: Take a moment to view yourself as an entity separate from your perspective. Reflect on your list of answers and meditate on this imagined version of yourself.

As humans, it's important to not only be self-aware and realize our choices in life but also recognize that others have unique ways of making choices. Just as I have my own approach to overcoming challenges, others do, too, and it's important to respect that. Similarly, while I may prefer one type of food, others may have different preferences, and that's okay. Ultimately, our choices in life should lead to acceptance and respect for one another. Have you experienced this before? If so, how did it go?

Dear Ibrahim,

Operations Technician in the Obstetrics and Pediatrics Department

I wanted to take a moment to express my gratitude for your support and guidance as a student in the Department of Obstetrics and Pediatrics. Your willingness to share your knowledge, time, and effort with us is greatly appreciated. I especially remember how you encouraged us to join the surgical skills program, which has been incredibly beneficial for us. I am also grateful for the book you shared with me as a reference. Your five books on the tools and basics of operations are some of the best and easiest to understand in the field. Thank you for your trust in us and for being a valuable member of our team.

Shampoo with Insecticide Extract!

Have you ever received a message on social media containing strange and fabricated tips embellished with many icons to draw attention? Some of these messages suggest using apple cider vinegar to burn belly fat or recommend not drinking cold water during meals to avoid transforming fat into a petroleum jelly-like substance. Others advise against trimming nails at night to avoid calcium deficiency. A postscript is often added to these messages to encourage reposting this information to benefit others. However, it's important to be cautious and fact-check before sharing information on social media.

I used to think that messages like these were only exchanged for fun and laughter. However, I stopped believing so after witnessing a disturbing case in the Paediatric Intensive Care Unit.

The atmosphere in the paediatric intensive care unit is

typically calm and focused, with routine procedures and continuous monitoring taking place. Nonetheless, this stability was suddenly disrupted when two nurses urgently brought in an eight-year-old girl who was struggling to breathe and had heart arrhythmia. It was initially unclear why she had been admitted as she was conscious and responsive to the doctor's inquiries. I approached to see a young child with a medium complexion, large eyes, and damp, thick hair. Despite her features, she seemed uneasy about the place and clung to her mother's cloak, repeating, "Mum, stay with me!" every few minutes. I attempted to greet them and inquire about the child's condition. Yet, when I saw the mother's tearful eyes and ulterior sense of remorse, I only offered comfort and monitored the child's vital signs. It was later discovered that the mother, who was sterilizing and disinfecting the pets in her home, followed one of the circulating rumours suggesting the use of pesticides to treat her daughter's head lice[(1)].

She mixed one of these pesticides with water and used it to

---

(1) Head lice are parasitic insects that can be found on the head, eyebrows, and eyelashes of people. Head lice feed on human blood several times a day and live close to the human scalp. There are types of lice that infect humans and others that infect pets.

wash her daughter's hair to kill lice or nits. The child suddenly had difficulty breathing, so the mother rushed to bring her to the hospital's emergency room. The medical staff quickly administered oxygen through a face mask and washed the child's hair to remove harmful chemicals. They then transferred her to the intensive care unit to monitor her vital signs and gave her smaller doses of medication to regulate her heartbeat and open up her airways. After some time, the child calmed down and was reassured. I was standing by myself, startled by the laughter that most staff held back. I couldn't understand how a rumour could be more potent than health awareness. Was the problem with the lack of health awareness or the strength of the rumour? I decided to investigate the source of rumours and found an informative article called "The Science of Rumours." According to the study, rumours are beliefs passed from person to person without evidence supporting validity. In 1940-1941, the first rumour about the occurrence of a second World War was recorded in American history, which took place in late 1941. This incident led experts to believe that people start rumours to stave off anxiety and fear. Psychologists Albert and Postman have formulated a concise yet insightful equation that explains the power of rumours. The law states that the significance of a rumour is based on the subject matter and the level of ambiguity surrounding it.

Rumour = importance of topic * level of ambiguity

When a subject matter holds significant importance for the audience, rumors surrounding it tend to be stronger and filled with ambiguous details. These details may include illogical analyses, like foreign words that were deliberately added or linking rumors to personal experiences or research. The reason for this is apparent, but we can fight against rumors and reduce their power by taking three simple steps. It is crucial that we don't blindly believe any information that we come across on social media without evidence to back it up. To ensure that we rely on reliable and official information, we should always refer to and verify the source of the information. Additionally, we must increase our basic scientific knowledge and develop critical thinking skills to evaluate any information we come across. This way, we can rely on our knowledge and thinking to guide us rather than relying on rumors to help us lose belly fat or trim our nails.

Dear Nurse Nour,

A Nurse in the Intensive Care Unit

I am much obliged to your deliberate steps, which are based on true scientific knowledge.

I will never forget when we discovered by chance that she registered to attend one of the preparation courses for the Saudi Commission for Health Specialties test with us, and when we asked her why she did that since she had passed this test a long time ago and was now an employee. She said her objective was to validate her medical information, nursing procedures, and developments in this area of science before applying them to the patient.

A Phantom of Pain!

For centuries, pain has been the top concern of scientists in general and health medical forces in particular. Nearly no hospital or unit is devoid of a pain complaint, whether primary or secondary chronic pain and all nursing care plans list reducing its severity as a chief objective. The Emergency Department is brimming with numerous patients who all share the feeling of pain that eventually led them to this department.

Moreover, the operating theatres echo with the moans and groans of patients after their recovery from surgery, as well as the cries of pain that come from delivery rooms announcing a new birth.

The cries of patients still resound in my ears, especially

those who are suffering from sickle cell anemia[1], we had come to expect to hear their cries every two hours of the day. These overwhelming cries, which are often mixed with imploring and pleading, cease only with the sedative injection that puts them in a deep sleep after all the procedures of care and attention fail to stop their pain. I also remember how a thirty-two-year-old patient squinted her eyes until the stabbing pain, which was caused by an abscess[2] in her right breast, faded away. Of course, I still recall the scene of an elderly patient digging her fingernails into the skin of my hand out of agonizing pain when the doctors removed a deep pressure ulcer[3] that occurred in her foot arch. I also witnessed other patients suffering all kinds of temporal and persistent pains that resided in their bodies.

---

(1) Sickle cell anemia is a common inherited blood disorder that causes our bodies to produce abnormally shaped red blood cells. The disease causes red blood cells to break down, resulting in pain attacks due to their accumulation in the blood vessels.

(2) An abscess is subcutaneous suppuration that leads to severe pain, which is usually caused by bacterial infections.

(3) The procedure of removing dead cells from a wound or ulcer, often using a surgical scalpel.

One patient, however, there is one patient who is still fresh in my memory and I still believe that he suffered the worst kind of pain I ever witnessed, even though I never heard his cries and he neither dug his nails into my hands nor squinted his eyes. He is one of the patients I encountered in the Psychological Health Clinic and had been suffering pain in a limb that was amputated years ago. The case was that he had painful sensations where his amputated toes were, even though it was a missing limb area now! It is medically known as phantom limb Pain[1]. It is often related to the remaining portion of the limb after amputation[2], where the pain sensation is often more severe close to the site of amputation than the amputated limb itself.

There is a difference between phantom pain, phantom sensation, and pain originating in the remaining part of the limb. While phantom pain is the patient's feeling of the presence of his amputated limb and the existence of pain in it, the phantom

(1) [edited by] Donna D. Ignatavicius, M. Linda Workman, Mary A. Mishler. Medical-Surgical Nursing across the Health Care Continuum, 2013, Pp. 1161.

(2) Nikolajsen L, Jensen TS. "Phantom Limb Pain," British Journal of Anaesthesia. 2001; 87: 107-116. Ketz AK.

sensation is the patient's feeling of the presence of his amputated part and the sense of numbness or tingling. As for the pain of the amputated limb, it is a pain that occurs due to amputation in the limb that precedes the site of amputation. Although the patient did not have a large part of his body amputated, his face was showing signs of depression as a result of this strange pain. He was pale and became so upset as he explained his condition. He even stopped going to work.

The underlying root cause of phantom pain is unclear yet, but there are efforts represented by several theories and experimental observations that attempt to explain what is going on. Some of them assume that tumors at the site of amputation might cause phantom pain, while others link it to the spinal cord and the lack of some elements in it, and some of them rely on the minute parts of the brain and monitoring them when pain occurs, and so on.

I have tried to think more divergently concerning this issue, and I do not intend to adopt what I say as a real cause; rather, I am trying to demonstrate my ideas about this pain. Therefore, I thought of causes nowhere near the theories about this issue. So, the cause could be, for example, a combination of the force of habit and mind activity. Probably, the mind used to activate several pain-inducing stimuli prior to the amputation of the limb, and it did not cease to do so after it was amputated.

Or why could not the cause be emotional and not physical pain? The BBC website published a study entitled: "Hurt Feelings' Worse than Pain'". The patient's feelings and his view of his physical appearance contribute a great deal to the process of his treatment. So, when this view is flawed, the pain may intensify by the remains of the amputated limb.

Was it a bad idea? Well, that is okay; a thinker once said, "You need a lot of bad ideas to come up with a few good ones."

Let's make another attempt! What about the fierce war taking place inside our bodies between the natural opioid analgesics that God created within our bodies at the base of our brains around the centers of pain, fear, and emotions on the one hand and pain triggers on the other hand? When the pain becomes chronic, analgesics withdraw, while when analgesics outmatch pain, they alleviate pain[(1)]. Perhaps pain triggers became accustomed to their

(1) Okasha, Ahmed. Physiological Psychology. Cairo, Dar Elmaref, 1986, Pp. 67.

place in the body part before its amputation so they accumulated in the remaining part and caused the patient to experience phantom pain.

As I reflected upon this phantom's mystery, I realized that nothing goes in vain inside our bodies because there is a reason and course for everything. Hence, I figured that it would be wise to put this concern out of my mind and wait for new theories by neuroscientists to appease my curiosity. Forget about my reflections. Do tell. What is the worst pain you have ever experienced?

Dear Dr. Saleh,

A dentist in a medical center

I appreciate that not a single patient leaves your clinic unless you restore one of his teeth or extract another.

I remember many patients who suffered tooth nerve pain, for instance, and although he would transfer them to another facility, he would examine their teeth thoroughly to point out another tooth that needed dental treatment. He is notable for his words: "I will restore this tooth so your visit to the clinic does not go in vain."

A Little Princess Inside the Hospital!

Once upon a time, after the Mesozoic Era, at dawn, the new morning sky was overcast with clouds and blazing with pink rays over friendly creatures hustling around. Welcome to the imagination world. Welcome to the Pediatric Hypnosis Clinic. One of the details that sparked my reflections and emotions the most was the cartoon characters that fill this section. They are on the doors of every room, patients' files, nurses' scrubs, and even my fingers, which I later tucked inside colorful clothing to keep up with this world. We have learned about the departments in this clinic and the nature of work there, and now it is time to meet the lovely inhabitants of this department.

We quietly pushed one of those doors to find a little creature, about a year and a half old, with eyes like pools of honey, small limbs, and a large head. He was suffering from hydrocephalus[1], which explains the swollen head, with a tube inserted surgically into a ventricle to drain excess fluid and reduce the pressure

Despite the buildup of fluid in his brain, which failed to distort his angelic features, the child was constantly quarrelsome and never tired of playing, and he naturally never stopped. As is the tendency of all children to play their spontaneous tricks and escape what they fear, he thus, ran away to hide his small body behind his mother, leaving us with no more than his smiling eyes.

After that, I sneaked into the next room... looking for a case that resembled my childhood and reminded me of myself at some point. It was neither this... nor that... oh! I found it.

A baby girl a few months old was in the middle of that bed, attached to the wall. She was born with three holes in her heart[2],

---

(1) Hydrocephalus is a condition characterized by an abnormal accumulation of cerebrospinal fluid within the ventricles (cavities) of the brain. It can cause babies and young children's heads to swell with convulsions and mental disorders.

(2) A hole in the heart is a type of congenital heart defect, and it may be an opening in the ventricular septum or the atrial septum of the heart. Its risk lies in that it affects the path of blood flow through the heart.

and no doubt that this explains the amount of love pouring into and from her. Two of them were plugged, but the third one failed to close on its own.

The child seemed to be in good health, and there was nothing to worry about in this condition, as the only risk was the flow of blood directly through that hole instead of passing through the main passages.

After introducing myself to the mother, I started looking through the file papers, hoping to understand the terms that did not seem intelligible to me at first glance because they were very adjacent. So, I started conversing with the mother and going through the file. Thus, I ended my day with thoughts and memories, comparing the procedures followed in my past with those followed in today's baby girl's case! I was born with the same defect in the heart but with only one hole, which naturally closed within time. However, the quaint thing about my interest in this case is that I have no memories of its effect. Rather, I only remember the monthly appointments, not much through the details of those appointments, but through the preparations before them, during which my parents excelled at creating a pleasant feeling to keep anxiety from overwhelming my frail heart. A few days before the appointment, my father used to pick me up to buy a new dress for my special date. Also, my mother used to fill the bathtub the night before to keep it warm and helped me take a shower, put on my dress, and do my hair. They were not preparing a patient going to the hospital with a feeling of defeat; rather, they were accompanying a little princess who would have her virtuous heart examined.

The appointment contained some disturbing details, such as the irritation associated with the pressure of the ultrasound scanner the doctor placed on my chest, the transparent gel ruining my clothes, and my long stay on that small bed. Yet, my mind was programmed to relate these appointments to cheerful details that were more profound and valuable. When I was informed about my next appointment, I forgot about all the annoying details, and my mind would rejoice at the sight of my new dress and my pleasant shower.

This was neither the first nor the last time that these memories came back to me; I also had flashbacks during a course that discussed scientific theories on mental and physiological health.

One of these theories was the "Little Albert" experiment, which was conducted by John Watson and Rosalie Rayner to show the possibility of applying the classical conditioning theory(1) to humans. They brought little Albert, who was 11 months old and introduced him to a friendly white rat.

With no prior fears, Albert spontaneously began touching the rat to express interest and curiosity. Watson then ordered to strike a steel bar with a hammer every time Albert tried to touch the mouse, and this was repeatedly done until the annoying sound was associated with the mouse. After that, as soon as the mouse was brought before Albert- without the annoying sound- Albert would be terrified and start crying. Not only that, but Albert also developed a fear of any furry animal or stuffed toy.

The annoying sound of the hammer against the steel bar may be resounding in a place crowded with white rats, and no one will care. Most of the tasks that should be handled may be associated with great deal unpleasant and good feelings all at once. The difference here is only convincing the mind or sometimes using

(1) Benson, Nigel, Joannah Ginsburg, and Voula Grand. The Psychology Book: Big Ideas Simply Explained. New York City, DK; First Edition, 2012.

children's tricks. This means that as long as our minds always show readiness to associate ideas, experiences, and feelings with each other, why can't we associate unpleasant tasks with good feelings to perform them and remember them later with a big smile and bright eyes? For example, my monthly appointments could be a source of resentment and result in psychological complexes and low self-esteem. However, they have been associated with the most beautiful gowns, so I looked forward to them. I even loved these appointments and ceased feeling embarrassed about them.

Therefore, when bad experiences are associated with good ideas, disturbing incidents turn into white clouds that pour good energy when you remember them later, and vice versa.

Note: I may not be authorized to give educational advice, but my appreciation and gratitude towards my parents when I remember my medical appointments are feelings worthy of being experienced by your children as well.

Dear Yousra,

The Anesthesia Technician in the Department of Pediatrics, Gynecology and Obstetrics

I just wanted to express my gratitude for the extra effort you put in to convince the patient to choose spinal instead of general anesthesia, not because it makes your job easier, but because it is a better option for the patient than having to endure the potential consequences of general anesthesia. I still remember how you took the time to speak with the patient before entering the operating room, providing a clear comparison between spinal and general anesthesia. This has always helped the patient feel reassured and make a well-informed choice.

Behind the Walls of Death

As we pursue success through constant hard work and learning, we may tread paths that steer us away from our intended route. Yet, lanes as such could be the narrow bridges that lead us to unfamiliar destinations. In these places, we will find people who strive to overcome their isolation and long to be embraced. By being heedful of any passerby, they anticipate being rescued by someone from the dreadful darkness that looms over them.

As I walk through these paths, I notice that many people here seem to be trapped in frustration and exhaustion due to serious illness that left them isolated and bedridden. The stillness of their isolation is only disrupted by the beeping sounds of medical equipment right here in the intensive care unit. I can hear a mechanical ventilator that acts as a bellow to move air in and out of the lungs, an electrocardiogram monitor recording vital signs such as blood pressure, pulse, breathing, and oxygen levels in the blood, and a blood purification apparatus carrying out the function of the kidneys. Additionally, the constant beeping sound of infusion pumps, which deliver nutrients and medications, may lessen the desolation of the place. Still, they could also add to the unit's overall tension.

As I watch the healthcare professionals who attend to these patients, I notice that doctors conduct quick examinations before performing a more thorough analysis. On the other hand, nurses provide medicinal supplies such as medications, nutrients, alimentary food, and cleaning equipment during their visits to the intensive care unit. Unfortunately, an uninvited guest lurks unnoticed sometimes, even in the presence of doctors and nurses; it is death! Although we all believe that death is inevitable and takes us to God's eternal resting place and His unconditional love, its sudden presence can be overwhelming and rigid, leaving us in a state of dread.

I recollect attending to a bedridden patient who never complained or talked but merely seized our hands as if she were communicating with us through her grip. She seemed to be yearning to convey her situation and say how her memories are gone with the wind. We expected her death since the beginning of that day. Therefore, a nurse had to accompany her in case of an emergency. I was next to her the whole time, recording her vital signs every ten minutes. Her vital signs showed that she was clinging to life; they were not entirely absent, so we could start resuscitating her, nor were they at their normal ranges. They were lower and slower than normal, similar in their pace to the drops of the intravenous drip hanging next to her. My emotions were so turbulent that I had to rush to the nurse whenever one of the values declined a degree or two to ensure whether or not it was normal.

Each time, she replied: "Wait! It is expected to decline more steeply!" Of course, this was not normal with all the medications, but it was to be expected for her present condition! I was distressed, and I believed it was negligence, but we knew deep down that the stages of death had begun, and one after another, the threads of her soul were deliberately slipping.

The second case that stood out was a cancer patient. It started in her right breast but then spread to her bones and liver, which caused the yellowing of her skin and the whites of her eyes.

She was resuscitated twice a day until she departed our world. I stepped in to help prepare and clean her to be taken to the morgue. Her chest was expanding and contracting because she was still on the mechanical ventilator, but as soon as we removed the endotracheal tube, her chest contracted at once. I was watching the top of her chest attentively to detect any possible indication of life in her body, but to no avail. When the nurse left for medical gauze, I stood alone with her. I felt a terrible sense of desolation that I looked away, unwilling to allow this feeling that weighed heavily on me to aggravate.

The third case was for a patient I attended to several times for a month. I saw her wrapped in a pale white cloth intended to shroud patients and then transfer them to the morgue. She suffered from brain stem bleed, which led to disorders in the functions it controls, such as movement, swallowing, and sometimes breathing. When the nurse told me that she had died early in the morning, I felt a lump in my throat as I stifled my tears and entered her room to check it. I advanced with shivering footsteps, bound where my feet took me, not where my will did. The patient's bed was placed in the corner of the room next to a large window, which allowed sunlight to penetrate the room as deeply as possible. This, all the more, made the room appear dimmer and darker to me, as if it contained thick, dense, dingy clouds that extended to the cheeks of her daughter, who sat on the bed by her side.

The last case was a deceased patient whose file was placed in the corner of the nurses' station table. It was tied in the middle with a strip of medical gauze to facilitate storing it in the old records repository where racks of files record the last moments of the lives of numerous people who mean a lot to their families. I picked up the first paper, which was the death certificate. It was pale green and jammed with handwritten notes that reached the margins: "The body of the patient whose identity is detailed above has been received and kept in the morgue."

I had vague emotions when experiencing all these details, something that I could not define. It was not fear, nor was it outright sadness. Prior to those feelings, with every case, I went through a denial stage. Every time I turned to my friends and said: "So fast! They declared that the patient was dead." My observation of vital signs and chest movement, my shivering feet, my reading of paper margins… All of my reactions indicated only one thing: I was in denial[(1)].

According to Dr. Elizabeth Kübler-Ross, a Swiss-American psychiatrist, denial is the first stage in a list of five stages of grief[(2)]. Unfortunately, these stages have been misinterpreted over the past decades and are considered a process of merely thrusting different emotional responses into an elegant order. However, the author finds that going through these emotions will help heal and alleviate the burden of grief, as many stories prove.

The five stages are denial, anger, bargaining, depression, and acceptance. Denial can be experienced by a person who is dying or those who have just experienced the loss of a loved one. People may experience all these stages in the suggested order, or they may experience one or some of them in a different order. When we encounter tragic life events like the ones I narrated, we may deny the reality of the situation as an attempt to convince ourselves that it is unreal and did not actually happen. This often

---

(1) The denial I felt was due to rejecting the sad event, not the idea of "death."

(2) Kubler-Ross, Elisabeth, and David Kessler. On Grief and Grieving. New York, Scribner, 2005, PP. 20-35.

leads to a frantic search for evidence to support our denial and seeking help from others to change this reality. This psychological defense mechanism is intended to shield ourselves from the intense emotions that come with accepting the truth. So, denying reality represents the inability to acknowledge it.

When we find that there is no way to deny it, our powers turn into anger when we realize that the situation is real. "Why me?" "What did I do to deserve all this?" and other angry, reproachful phrases might be our way to verbalize this anger. The expressions of anger need not be logical or correct; we release them to calm our anger, not to get answers. This anger may be triggered by several reasons: we either feel angry at the deceased person because they did not take care of themselves and consequently died abandoning us, or angry at ourselves because we did not care enough to protect them from death, or because we did not spend more time with them when they were around, or we may be angry at ourselves because we could not prevent their death!

Anger often leads our way towards emotions like sadness, panic, and loneliness. We may try to find ways to delay the loss of a loved one, entering into a stage of bargaining. During this stage, we replay past events and wonder what could have been done differently. However, we must come to accept the fact that our loved one is gone.

Then, we become conscious of our grief and find ourselves in a state of depression. This grief may be so deep that we feel it will never dissipate, and we have disconnected from life. We become consumed by the thick fog of sadness and apathy, which makes us bedbound. It's important to recognize that this experience is not a psychological disorder but a natural response to losing a loved one. These five stages of grief are significant in the healing process, and it's essential to acknowledge and embrace them. Eventually, we will become conscious of our emotions and learn to live with them.

There comes a time when we must accept reality and find solace in coming to terms with it. It's crucial to understand that accepting does not necessarily mean feeling positive sentiments regarding the loss of a loved one. Instead, it is about accepting their departure and confronting the truth of their absence. We probably face difficulties in accepting this reality, but acknowledging it can assist us in overcoming grief instead of prolonging it. What I was experiencing when each patient died fits the profile of these psychological stages. Because loved ones will eternally exist in our souls, these stages may expand until we end up living with the last stage, which is always remembering our happy moments with the deceased and constantly praying for them.

May almighty God have mercy on them, grant them eternal peace, and place their souls in heaven.

Dear Ibrahim,

A nurse in the emergency department,

I would like to express my gratitude for your ardent care for the patient beneficence.

I remember when a patient was lying on the bed with low blood pressure, and nurse Ibrahim was persistently arguing with the doctors that patients' rights and respect should be a priority.

I also recall the day when his face was pale, and he kept drinking coffee all day. Later, I found out that he had been working through the night shift and had already completed a workday but chose to stay to help others. He worked for 16 hours nonstop that day.

God is the Best of Inheritors

God Almighty says in the Holy Quran: "O My Lord, leave me not alone (without an heir). And you are the best of inheritors[1]."

As you walk past the maternity and children's hospitals in the area, you will notice this verse on one of the walls that leads to the delivery rooms. Take a moment to reflect on its meaning, for there is no better place to do so.

I have always pondered on this verse as I encountered it wherever I would turn. This time, I was assigned to attend to patients in the maternity emergency department. Here, mothers arrive experiencing varying pains, unaware of what awaits them, until the doctors decide that they need to go into labour immediately. They endure overwhelming pains and weariness but

(1) (Al Quran – The Prophets, 21:89)

finally rejoice at the arrival of their new-borns, witnessing God's precious gift to them.

Unfortunately, not all mothers exit the delivery room feeling happy. At times, they lose their fetuses at birth, and they exit suppressing their emotional pain along with their tears and cries; and sometimes, they may come out after they have departed our world forever.

Giving birth is, undoubtedly, one of the most significant experiences any mother can have in her lifetime. It involves not just physical but also mental exertion. Any sudden deterioration in the mother's condition can pose a threat to the life of her child, her own life, or both. Therefore, she must quickly decide to address the situation and avoid any life-threatening risks.

I recall a popular story circling around the hospital, narrated by one of the nurses. It was about a patient who, after trying to conceive for so long, was finally blessed by God with twins. So ecstatic the mother was that she eagerly counted down the days until she could finally see her babies. At the time of labour, she was told that a cesarean section was the best option for the twins.

However, she decided to try having a natural birth, even if it was only for a few minutes.

As time passed, the fetuses' health declined, which posed a threat to their lives. The medical staff decided to transfer her to the operating room, and all they needed was the guardian's approval.[1], but he refused. The husband believed that his wife was capable of giving natural birth, alluding to the mothers and grandmothers who delivered in their homes decades ago.

Despite the efforts made by the doctor and the medical staff to reach out to the mother's family to no avail, they could not resolve this, even after explaining the complications that could possibly lead to death. It was only minutes before the mother and her twins passed away. Whether this story is true or not, or if it is a mere fabrication, I am positive that incidents as such commonly happen, not solely in the operating theatre but in the theatre of the real world as well. So, what are the reasons for making a wrong decision?

---

(1) According to the nurse, this story happened back in the old days, but a new policy is followed at the present in emergency cases, where the mother herself or several doctors are allowed to sign in case of an emergency.

In his book, *Decision Making*, Dr. Sherif Shehata explains that the reasons for making wrong decisions can be summed up in nine points:

1- Incorrect reading of the situation: "This is directly caused by insufficient information and realistic assessments, which means that the decision may be delayed or not even made lest it be a hasty one[(1)]." To overcome this point, we can pose questions using five keys: why, what, where, when, and who.

2- The lack of available alternatives: That is the deliberate choices. The more available deliberate choices there are, the more well-rounded the decisions tend to be. Thus, the individual's tendency to be biased for a particular decision is determined by the number of deliberate choices available.

3- Acting impulsively and ignoring the facts: Here, the individual chooses what they desire and what they like without considering the consequences.

4- Disorganization and confused priorities: If a person is

(1) Shehata, Sherif. Decision Making. Giza, Dar Al Raya, 2016, Pp.19.

confused about their priorities, they end up making the wrong choices due to their inability to determine what is important to them. For instance, they fail to determine whether their money or well-being comes first.

5- Financial barriers: Just as money may be one of our priorities, it could also be an obstacle that stands in the way of making the right decision.

6- Amplifying the decision-making process: An aura of anxiety surrounds the decision-making process, catastrophizing its outcome and blurring our vision of the right decision.

7- Expecting a random outcome: It means a lack of seriousness of the decision and a lack of responsibility towards it.

8-The timing of the decision and external influences: This is one of the reasons the mother mentioned above faced. Of course, weighing our alternatives to choose the correct ones will not be the best way when the decision is to be made urgently. Moreover, external influences can hinder our selection process, as humans are naturally inclined to feel reassured when they share the same tendencies with their loved ones, especially when struggling with a challenge that must be dealt with within a limited time frame.

Our lives are shaped by a series of decisions that we make every day, some of which are simple, while others are immediate and can be life-changing. Any step forward or backward, each decision we make has a significant impact on our lives. Therefore, eliminating the causes of poor decision-making raises the likelihood of effective decision-making.

Dear mother, when you pack your hospital bag for delivery, do not forget to include alternative plans and possibilities and make decisions, even if tentative, regarding them. And God is the best of inheritors.

Dear Mohamed,

The Surgical Technician in the Department of Pediatrics, Gynecology, and Obstetrics,

You have my heartfelt gratitude for your guidance in mastering even the most basic details. I still remember how vexed you were when I inadvertently used a white medical gauze on a wound that was stained with Povidone-iodine solution.

Where Do the Ideas Hide?

I started my morning at a primary healthcare rehabilitation centre in a small room with three beds separated by sheer curtains, as still as the patients lying behind them. These patients were fatigued and bored due to prolonged bed rest and immobilization. The air was thick with loud silence, with only the monotonous rhythm of my breathing to break it.

I was observing a patient in the autumn of his life whose memory loss left him confused and unable to recognize the faces of those around him. He occasionally fell into a deep sleep and awoke to bask in the warm sunlight streaming through the window.

Suddenly, I heard finger snaps from the bed on my far right. A recording of a melodious prayer began to play, filling the room with a spiritual essence. I listened to the prayer with the other person in the room, who was two beds away from me. I waited for the prayer to end to speak with him before he fell asleep.

About half an hour passed before the appointment for physical therapy. Then, I learned that he was that patient who lived to watch the progressive degeneration of his muscles before his eyes. First, it began developing in his lower limbs, feet, legs, and thighs, and now the disease is trying to eat away at his right hand, and he is trying to resist it with physiotherapy sessions. He suffers from multiple sclerosis[(1)], a disease that strikes without warning or reason, like a recurring nightmare. The physiotherapist greeted the patient warmly, for they had known each other for a long time. He started the session by focusing on the patient's feet in a futile attempt to bring them back to life.

As the doctor worked with the patient, they engaged in a conversation I could not initially hear. Shortly, however, I was astounded to overhear that their discussion was about the Big

---

(1) Multiple sclerosis is a condition that affects the central nervous system and disrupts the brain's ability to send and receive signals. The symptoms and signs of this illness, include both organic and cognitive mental symptoms, as well as psychological problems.

Bang Theory[1], rather than just the progress in the patient's case. I had assumed that their discussion would only revolve around the patient's health, so this was unexpected.

What surprised me even more was that the discussion did not follow the classical Socratic Tradition of argumentative dialogue between individuals assuming a right and false side.

The debate was held in a competitive atmosphere rather than a neutral discussion. Each participant tried to complete the picture, lending a fresh perspective to the subject. The patient was alluding to Quranic verses, which made me realize his interest in spiritual matters. As much as I enjoyed listening to the smooth discussion, I eagerly waited for its end so that I could have a conversation with the patient.

When I had the opportunity to speak, I introduced myself as the assigned training student in the room. The patient looked sorrowful and dejected, which was only to be expected given that

(1) The Big Bang theory suggests that the universe began from an extremely hot, dense point smaller than a subatomic particle. An unimaginable force caused the intense burst of energy from the tiny point in a fraction of a second distributing all the matter and energy in all directions.

dealing with the same tedious details daily made him feel stuck in a huge chasm separating the soul from the whole world.

However, I decided to lift his sorrow by engaging him in a conversation about his interest in spiritual matters. “It is worthy of admiration to look at things from different points of view,” I said. “Like how you lend a spiritual perspective to the discussion. Have you ever tried contemplating the Qur’an? Perhaps by thinking deeply on one verse each day?” I asked. I then pointed out that many people are devoted to memorizing the Qur’an, but rarely does anyone take the time to contemplate it. My words came spontaneously to steer our conversation in another direction. His reaction, though, was surprising to me. He remained silent momentarily, smiled, and asked, “What else?” I suddenly felt a rush of heat in my body that settled in my head. I was overwhelmed with fear that his unexpected response would be a prelude to harsh words I would not want to hear. “I am a little confused,” I replied. “What else?” He was simply asking me to elaborate. I breathed a sigh of relief and expatiated on the subject for the duration of my work hours. When I left, he was smiling, with his eyes fixed downwards, and I hoped that he was thinking about our talk.

As I began my duties the following day, as soon as I entered the room and greeted him as usual, he promptly said, as if waiting for me to come: "Our talk left me thinking about so many things." I felt a burst of vitality and positive energy! In a sudden epiphany, I realized that there is nothing more valuable than spurring someone to think, regardless of how much moral or material support you offer them.

"Taking plants as an example," he proceeded, "some of them exhibit human-like traits such as sensations or meat consumption. Additionally, when considering the motion of celestial bodies, it was recently discovered that there are twelve planets, not eight, which means four additional planets. How will they discover them, and when will it happen? And where could they be? Moreover, what about the building blocks of matter? You know, now they have discovered an additional state of matter known as plasma, but there is no clear explanation. There are so many other things to contemplate."

I am amazed and smiling as it is my turn to listen to his speech. I find it remarkable how he can gather such vast amounts of information and keep up with the latest scientific breakthroughs. I wonder how he could draw this information about various subjects like plants, animals, and astronomy. Were these thoughts always within him? What prompted him to express these ideas? Where have these ideas been hiding all along? This is why Kevin Dunbar, a professor of psychology, was interested in investigating scientists generating new ideas through visiting four molecular biology laboratories and conducting naturalistic observations of scientists in their labs. He recorded videos of workers from different angles inside the laboratories during his visits. He observed them while they were examining slides under microscopes with excitement and anticipation of discovery. Dunbar also observed their casual conversations in the hallways that reinforced their feelings of belonging and their weekly gatherings around the conference table, where they shared a common interest and passion.

Over the course of four years he spent in the alleys of these laboratories, he discovered the secret hideout where most ideas are collected. Out of the three places he observed, which place do you think has the most ideas?

It is the conference room where the weekly gatherings take

place. We often think of the conference room as a dull and uneventful space. Yet, it is the perfect place to spur creativity and ideas. This is why the mind of my educated patient was overflowing with various ideas at once. Having someone to share your ideas and interests fosters an environment that nurtures the growth of ideas to flourish within you, granting you the liberty to pursue them in whatever direction you please. In order to draw out new ideas from your imagination, seek out the ideal environment to do so, starting with the perfect group or individual.

I am uninformed of the progress made in the patient's condition presently, but I hope he will always be well and never stop thinking.

Dear Maryam,

The Respiratory Therapist in the Intensive Care Unit

I would like to say thank you for your commendable attention to every detail in your work. While everyone struggles with their work tasks, it is impressive how nimbly you move from one patient to another to ensure that everything is taken care of.

Which Question Shall I Start with?

A new day has begun, and morning sunbeams are gently floating in the ceiling to weave a new sky above the calm room. The silence in the room was interrupted by the tumult of the medical staff as part of their morning routine.

This time, I decided to join the physiotherapy therapy session of the educated patient, as yesterday's conversation increased my desire to know more about the details and implications of his illness.

When the therapist came, I expressed my desire to accompany him, to which he agreed. I was worried that my presence might cause some discomfort to the patient. However, any such concerns were quickly dispelled as the doctor and the patient began to discuss the disease that was invading his frail body. The patient fell silent as the doctor persisted in explaining in detail the various symptoms, such as defects of vision, paraesthesia, weakness in the lower extremities, and a possible loss of the ability to walk independently or ambulate at all. The doctor also emphasized the importance of physical therapy and medications to prevent further relapses. At the end of his speech, the patient said something that concerned me. He spoke in a broken tone with sorrow: "There is no need to be embarrassed, doctor!" The doctor replied, "Why embarrassment? We are discussing the disease like any other, and we did not discuss your personal details!" I took a deep breath and found nothing more appropriate than silence to soothe the situation and console the patient.

It is such an excruciating pain for a person to face the very details they are trying to avoid! In a moment of introspection, I lowered my head and noticed the book I had brought. It was about the brain and its development based on modern research.

I saw this as an opportunity to share my interest in the subject. I said, "Ever since my studies, I have been fascinated by neuroscience and the brain's anatomy."

"Neurology is a multidimensional science," the doctor replied.

When talking about nerves, we have to consider various aspects - their anatomy, vital functions, integrative networks with the brain regarding signalling, and the brain's cognitive and social functions." I smiled with enjoyment at sharing my interests with someone more knowledgeable than yourself to enlighten you and broaden your horizon.

The doctor moved to the patient's right hand and held his palm in the shape of a fist, alternating it up and down. I then explained: "What makes neuroscience challenging is the vast array of possibilities and the inability to identify the primary causes of most illnesses." "Right!" The doctor agreed: "Multiple sclerosis is a perfect example of this. There are several theories regarding the possible etiologies of this disease. Some suggest that what triggers the risk factors include a viral infection, family history, reduced cerebrospinal fluid, and a sedentary lifestyle."

Our discussion provoked the patient into conversation, and he finally spoke to reveal a valuable lesson that I added to the list of insights gained from patients. The lesson was simple yet profound: "Always start with (how) something happened, and you will end up discovering (why) it happened!" I appreciated the wisdom in this statement and began projecting it to various aspects of my life, and each time, his lesson proved to be of invaluable help.

We may always wonder: (why) we fail to achieve our goals, and we disregard the question of (how) we pursue these goals.

So, perhaps instead of exhausting ourselves with the question: (Why) did I flunk my exams? The right question to ask is: (How) did I prepare for my exam?

When we learn to build critical thinking skills through coordinating intellectual efforts in ascending order, we start with remembering, then understanding, and move on to the higher levels of applying, analyzing, and evaluating. At the top of the pyramid, there is creating. Each level has a specific guiding question. In the initial stages of remembering and understanding, the question asked is usually "How?" On the other hand, the higher levels of applying, analyzing, evaluating, and creating are designated with the question of "Why?"

I found that my patient's words followed this path of

questioning, which shows how important it is to ask the right questions at each level of critical thinking.

If you want to think critically about a problem, there is a scientific order that can be followed. First, you should recall and remember the relevant information, then try to understand it by asking (how) it happened. Next, you can start applying this information and analyzing the results while keeping in mind the question of (why) it happened. By evaluating the information and understanding its causes, you can repeat the process of application and analysis until you reach the stage of creativity. Through this process, you can gain a clear understanding of the issue at hand and develop novel solutions. If we assume that thinking skills are arranged in the shape of a pyramid, then "how" will be at the base of the pyramid, leading to "why" at its top. Both the base and the summit are complementary, as there are no foundations without bases and no complementarity without summits.

Tell me now: Was I mistaken when I said that he was an "educated patient"?

Dear Dr. Hussein,

An Anesthesiologist in the Division of General Surgery

I wanted to express my gratitude for taking the time to thoroughly understand the medical history of each case before handling it. Initially, I assumed you were an intensive care doctor due to the amount of time you spent reviewing patients' files. However, I later learned that you are an anesthesiologist in the operating department who dedicates time to reviewing the files of cases scheduled for surgery.

Our Basic Needs

The chirping of sparrows, gentle breeze, and glistening dewdrops heralded a new morning. I was assigned to work at the Occupational Therapy Center[(1)] of the Mental Health Hospital, where the patients engage in creative activities. The center comprised four sections, namely, the drawing room and a workshop where the residents created beautiful works of art despite their neutral symptoms. I was always fascinated by their art creations, which equally included implicit and explicit details. From the intricate frames to the lines and shapes, their works had a unique spirit and were often sold at the hospital's outdoor events.

(1) Occupational therapy is one of the support medical professions that is based on assessing patients to treat them by training them in daily life skills.

Within the facility, there is also a sewing studio equipped with embroidery and decoration tools. Patients have the opportunity to learn how to sew and create their pieces, which inspires them to pursue their hopes and dreams.

The last section is the computer room, which is equipped with computers to teach patients basic skills. The last section is a classroom where lessons and counseling are provided to patients.

Stable patients are hosted in the facility, and their stability is measured by their lack of setbacks and any attempts to harm themselves or others. The Occupational Therapy Centre is visited by the same group of patients every day until they become accustomed to the place and almost feel bored. They begin to see no difference between the facility and their rooms in the Inpatient Care Unit. Within this center, patients have the opportunity to refresh their memory which has become inactive by embracing the same daily details to the point that each of them has come to expect everything before it happens, not because she has supernatural powers in reading minds, but by the power of repetition and monotonous routine.

There were four patients diagnosed with schizophrenia[1], but they had unique psychological attributes. The only commonality among them was episodic, recurrent hallucinations. One of the patients had been staying in the Inpatient Department for more than two decades. Her psychological state had deteriorated to the point that it made her adapt to her condition and live with what was happening to her as if it were the natural way of living.

During our conversation, she perceived many auditory hallucinations[2] and seemed to respond to both of us in a strange harmony, which merely bothered her instead of frightening her. Similarly, the second patient had a long stay in the hospital, but her condition is different. Although she was able to choose her words and facial expressions naturally, in a way that corresponded to the content of her speech, the symptoms of schizophrenia occasionally affected her. She experienced sudden changes in perception, such as mistaking daytime for nighttime. We used to

(1) Schizophrenia is a chronic brain disorder, characterized by thoughts or experiences that seem out of touch with reality and disorganized social behavior.

(2) Auditory hallucinations are sensory perceptions of hearing in the absence of an external stimulus.

call the third patient, the poet and advisor, for she used to stand tall and recite poetry verses about different instances and people, offering advice on various topics. The fourth patient was the shyest and most reserved among these patients, and her shyness prevented her from participating in many activities.

Our task in the Occupational Therapy Center was to entertain the patients. Hence, we attempted to test their memory with intuitive tasks and assess their movability and the negative impact that medicine adverse effects had on them. The patients' interactions were successful, especially the fourth patient who showed noticeable changes in her interaction, movement, and overcoming shyness. After several cognitive-motor interventions, it was time to give the patients a time-out to practice their favorite activities individually. Some favored drawing, others preferred walking, and some liked to practice dancing.

We occasionally walked around the patients and sat with them every now and then.

It came to my notice that the fourth patient had stopped drawing a while ago. So, I approached her and suggested going for a walk outside, and she agreed. Hearing the gentle rustling of trees and feeling the freshness of the earth, added to the pleasantness and intimacy of the atmosphere. I deliberately remained silent, hoping that the patient herself would lead the conversation. After a few minutes of silence, she suddenly said: "I have four sisters and five brothers." She listed their names in descending order and then asked: "What about you?" I answered her with apparent interaction and simple details, but her question occupied a large part of my thoughts that day.

The patient was not logically driven to put a question as such, nor did she carefully choose it from a fleeting conversations list. Rather, she allowed her soul to speak up and took refuge in her safest haven to share her thoughts. Being surrounded by family members, having a home, belonging, and feeling loved, are all basic psychological needs. Despite our differences, we all pursue these needs consciously or unconsciously in diverse ways.

Abraham Maslow, a specialist in analytical psychology, made observations of the patients who visited his clinic and concluded that innate human needs unconsciously drive human actions and behaviors. According to Maslow, people automatically pursue the satisfaction of these needs, but the approach and extent of satisfaction differ from one person to another.

Maslow also suggests that the hierarchal order, according to which individuals fulfill these needs, is associated with the individual's adaptation to their surroundings and circumstances.

So, what are these basic needs?

The pyramid of basic needs comprises five levels. The lower level is the physiological needs or biological requirements for human survival

that include breathing, water, air, food, and sleep. The second level is the need for security and safety, which is the need to live within a stable and organized environment, free from any material or moral threats. After physiological and safety needs have been fulfilled, the third level of human needs is social and involves feelings of love and belongingness. It refers to a human emotional need for interpersonal relationships, affiliating, connectedness, and being part of a group.

The fourth level is the need for self-esteem, which includes self-worth, accomplishment, and the individual's need to feel respected and valued by others.

The fifth and highest level in Maslow's hierarchy is the need for self-actualization, which refers to the full exploitation of a person's potentialities and talents, self-fulfillment, seeking personal growth, and peak experiences. It can be described as the desire to develop to the full stature of which one is capable.

Maslow categorized human needs into two main types: deficiency needs and growth needs. The former includes the lower-order three needs, namely physiological needs, the need for security, and the need for love and belonging. If these needs are not adequately met, it can hinder the individual's physical and psychological growth.

On the other hand, growth needs or higher-order, such as the need for self-esteem and self-actualization. Meeting these needs corresponds to a person's self-fulfillment, personal growth, and attaining the level of human perfection.

When one of these needs is satisfied, a new (and "higher") need emerges to become salient and dominate the individual.

Unfortunately, the progress up the hierarchy is at times disrupted by a failure to meet lower-level needs. It is a fact that the more a person can address higher needs, the more they boost their mental health and achieve self-fulfillment[1].

Conversely, many studies conducted on children in social institutions who did not receive love and feel belongingness had shown that their growth was not normal despite addressing their physiological needs within those institutions.

To apply Maslow's hierarchy of needs to our lives, we can simply envision an ideal life and observe how these needs align. The basic physiological needs, such as food, sleep, and oxygen, occupy the lower level. Once these innate needs are satisfied, we can proceed with a vigorous mind and a full stomach to fulfill other needs. We unconsciously seek security in various aspects of our lives, including work, financial stability, and resource acquisition, such as affording a roof to feel safe. Once this need is addressed, we proceed to look for a sense a sense of belonging and love by affiliating ourselves with a group family and friends.

---

(1) Engler, Barbara. Personality Theories: An Introduction. Pennsylvania, Houghton Mifflin, 1985.

After becoming part of a group, we strive for distinction to gain recognition, confidence, and self-esteem and to achieve self-actualization, where creativity, innovation, and support for others can thrive.

I wonder if my patient's question suggested a deeper concern! Was she seeking a sense of belonging to move on to a higher-order need?

Dear Nurse Zahra,

A nurse in the Intensive Care Department

I am grateful for the excellent guidance and structured education you provided. Your daily list of the topics we would cover was very helpful. Your willingness to go above and beyond was truly inspiring. I noticed that your dedication was not limited to interns like myself. I have seen you, at times, patiently explain to staff nurses how to operate one of the existing devices and repeat the explanation to us as well.

And Then What?

The night has fallen, and it is now time for me to close my eyes and drift off to sleep. However, I am finding it difficult to do so as my mind is cluttered with thoughts and tasks that need to be completed. This reminds me of a poem by Layth al-Sandouq, who wrote about how we often forget things amidst the chaos of our lives:

"In the busyness of life, we tend to forget the faces of those who left on a train.

We forget the paths over which our jaded eyes had lingered very long.

We forget our names carved on the tree boles that bear our memories.

Amidst the desperate chaos, we forget the faces that once

shone like lanterns in the darkness of our lives.

We forget the eyes that once chiseled the walls of our despair.

We forget the hands that once wiped away our tears.

Amidst the chaos, we may shut out the light of the world around us by building walls around our eyes.

We may sacrifice our own solace, ripping the hearts out of our chests to feed the whales,

and in doing so, leave our loved ones stranded in a sinking boat, struggling in the lake of oblivion."

I woke up and recited these verses to myself, creating a mental barrier preventing the outside world's chaos from overwhelming me. Until I ended up reading the same verses in the eyes of a patient who seemed to be a lost soul. It was not the busyness of life that made him fade into oblivion, but rather the void he felt inside.

Here, at the Rehabilitation and Palliative Care Center, patients with various diagnoses but similar medical needs require basic care due to their inability to carry out daily tasks. The center is divided into two sections: the women's ward and the men's ward. Each section has a small area in the middle, surrounded by small patient rooms. The area is well-lit, with natural light streaming through large glass windows. The patient rooms house three to four beds each and cater to patients who require assistance with mobility.

I made a conscious effort to avoid the men's ward at work as I was afraid of being assigned to one of the rooms there. I was specifically worried about being placed in the corner room, which housed a patient with strange behaviors. This thirty-nine-year-old man would attempt to get the attention of or engage in conversation with anyone who passed by, even though his speech was often slurred. When the chief nurse noticed that many of us shared the same fear, she explained his condition to us.

When this patient was seventeen, he and his friend challenged each other in a street drag race. They were young, impulsive, and reckless. They did not make the slightest effort to reconsider their decision, nor did they choose the right track, time, or procedure.

They started the race with great excitement and loud laughter, but as the end drew near, his friend disappeared along with everyone else. The patient found himself alone behind the steering wheel of his car, heading at a crazy speed down a dark, unpaved road. Because the road was rugged, his car collided and crashed. He finished the race alone and continued on his own. He suffered a serious traumatic brain injury and remained in a coma for three years, which disrupted the normal functions of his brain and, subsequently, the functions of other organs.

It wasn't as painful as remembering the details of the accident three years later, after waking up from a coma with both legs and one hand disabled.

He could remember the details of the accident as if it had happened yesterday. Not only that, he was waiting for his friend to come check on him, but he never came.

A story like this was sufficient to make me forget about everything occupying my mind and break off what was going on in my day, forcing me to focus on it. I did not ruminate about his medical condition, nor did I reflect on his bad company. Instead,

I found myself wondering: Why do harmful behaviors as such still persist? Unfortunately, this story is not the first of its kind. We all have heard similar stories about people being victimized by reckless behavior. So, what drives this behavior and why do people keep practicing it?

Burrhus Frederic Skinner, an American psychologist, was interested in human behavior, especially how unplanned behaviors shape and the various factors and motivations that reinforce them. Thus, he created the term "operant conditioning [(1)]" and codified its basic principles. He suggested the best way to understand human behavior is to look at the causes of action along with its negative and positive consequences. Skinner believed that the reinforcements that follow a certain action are of greater influence than the stimuli that precede it. In other words, the outcomes that result after the occurrence of a behavior may contribute to the perpetuation of that behavior more than the influences that come prior to its occurrence.

He considered this a condition associated with our behaviors

(1) Benson, Nigel. The Psychology Book: Big Ideas Explained. DK Publishing, London, 2011, Pp. 78.

and actions in life. After conducting experiments on mice in a small box, Skinner published his theory, dividing the motivations associated with a behavior into incentives and punishments, or reward and punishment.

Before delving into details to clarify his ideas, we should ask ourselves: What drives us to do something? Is it the promise of a reward or the fear of punishment? What motivates us: the carrot or the stick? Let's find out together.

Skinner classified stimuli into two types: rewards and punishments. A reward strengthens a behavior, making it more likely to be repeated. On the other hand, a punishment weakens a behavior, decreasing the likelihood of repeating it. Ultimately, it is up to us to choose whether or not to practice a certain behavior based on the associated rewards or punishments.

Stimuli that reinforce behavior can be categorized into two types: positive reinforcers and negative reinforcers[(1)].

A positive reinforcer strengthens the behavior by presenting a

(1) Positive and negative do not mean good or bad. Rather, positive means adding something, and negative means removing something.

positive stimulus, which motivates the individual. In other words, we engage in a particular behavior for the desirable outcome that follows it. For instance, the patient might have suggested a race to his friend (behavior), driven not by the intense adrenaline rush they would get but by the good feelings triggered by winning and receiving admiration from his friend or simply to have a good laugh (positive reinforcer). In this case, the positive outcome serves as a reinforcement for the behavior.

A negative reinforcer, on the other hand, involves the removal of unfavorable events or outcomes after the display of a behavior. In these situations, a response is strengthened by the removal of something considered unpleasant. This means that an individual's action leads to the removal of the unpleasant condition, negatively reinforcing their behavior. For example, when the patient suggested the race to his friend, he would fasten the seat belt (behavior) not to abide by traffic laws but to avoid a collision (an undesirable outcome). In this case, avoiding the negative outcome serves as a reinforcement for the behavior.

Similarly, there are two kinds of punishment: positive and negative. In both of these cases, the behavior decreases. **Positive**

punishment is when we avoid a certain behavior because we are afraid of getting punished later. For instance, the patient may refuse the race (behavior) not because he does not want it but to avoid getting a traffic ticket for a driving offense which stands for the removal of an unfavorable outcome.

Negative punishment, however, is when we avoid a certain behavior in order not to lose something that we like. For example, the patient may refuse the race (behavior) not because he does not want it but to avoid risking his well-being in a traffic accident, which stands for the removal of a favorable outcome.

Skinner's theory suggests that we can limit our random unplanned behaviors by being aware that a reckless action would lead to an unpleasant result, and by avoiding that action, we redeem our self-respect. Namely, all these theories can be encapsulated in one question we should ask ourselves each time we intend to take an action: "And then what?" This would help us identify potential disincentives and consequences and, therefore, decide to refrain from certain behaviors or venture upon them, or perhaps it could be too late to ask any questions!

The chief nurse saw that the patient's story justified his attention-seeking behavior and believed that it was his way to maintain his health and well-being so that he would not succumb to the states of despair and frenzy he had repeatedly experienced.

He was possibly engaging in a behavior that was instilled as a result of a prior punishment. Unfortunately, in his attempts to communicate with us, he may have been pleading for answers to the question "Then what?" after that ship had sailed long ago.

Dear Operation Theater Technician Ahmed,

The Department of Pediatrics, Gynecology and Obstetrics

I would like to thank you for promoting reinforcement learning in the workplace. Even during the most dramatic moments, you never miss an opportunity to reinforce and acknowledge our successful work, even if it was spontaneously done.

Emotions: Do they govern us or do we govern them?

Each day, we wake up from the warmth of dreams, which fade away as soon as we are faced with the coldness of reality. Time covers the present moment, and we delve into the depths of life amidst the clamor of our various tasks and the emotions associated with them. We live in a series of moments without realizing their cohesion and continuity until something disrupts this flow and sheds light solely on the moment, turning the present upside down. "When did this case start?" My thoughts were interrupted by the doctor's question to a man in his thirties who came with his elderly mother to the emergency room at the mental health hospital. The man entered the room with his mother, filled with fear for her. He whispered to the staff, revealing his tricks to convince her to come. The seventy-year-old woman calmly listened to the doctor's routine questions and answered them in detail and with good interaction. There was nothing wrong with the woman. Rather, she displayed unparalleled prudence and kindness, but it was necessary to diagnose the alleged sickness. It did not take long to show its symptoms, exactly in my arms.

She suddenly began complaining about the dwarfs who wandered about, trying to enrage her by causing chaos everywhere, even inside the food dishes. Now they're all over her, jumping into her arms. She tried to disperse them with her hand at times and with her angry words at others.

The doctor realized that she was undoubtedly experiencing a visual hallucination and began to write her notes while asking a good number of questions to the son to reach the correct diagnosis for her condition: "When did this condition begin?" The son replied: "After my brother's death." The doctor stopped writing because his words could change her report and the possible diagnosis. "My brother died a few months after my father's death. He had been suffering from cancer for a long time, but he kept it from all of us. On the day he was supposed to travel for treatment, he told us about it right before we said goodbye. Unfortunately, he died before he made it to the airport.

My mother was overwhelmed with grief and began to see those imaginary dwarfs.

From the complexities of aging, my thoughts move to the simplicity of childhood, to that naughty seven-year-old child. His father complained about his recklessness and how he gets into trouble without thinking! The father was infuriated by the dangerous games his child played; his heedless way of using tools and even throwing himself in front of the cars was all infuriating. This was evident as the child was hyperactive, fidgety, restlessly turning around, and constantly shaking his feet.

The doctor diagnosed the boy with an intellectual disability and began to justify the boy's behavior accordingly. He asked the father to bring the papers designated for preparing a medical record audit to fill out and quickly move on to the next patient. The record included routine questions asked to the patient by the doctor, such as, "Do you hear anyone talking to you in your ear or see anyone?" The doctor was about to write a negative answer to the question when the boy replied, "Yes, I hear something." His answer left everyone confused. "Who do you hear?" the doctor asked in amazement. "I hear my uncle's voice speaking to me." His father's eyes misted over as he tried his best to clear up our confusion. He explained that his son's condition did not exacerbate until he saw his uncle killed in front of him! "How did he see his uncle killed?" the doctor inquired.

"They called me from the train station and said that I had to come urgently. Unfortunately, I took my boy with me. I did not expect that it would be about a murder and that there was a corpse. A lot of people gathered there, and we were surprised to see my brother lying on the ground killed. My boy was next to me and witnessed everything."

The room was suddenly quiet, and we were trying hard to figure out the correct diagnosis for that innocent child. The doctor pursed his lips, expressing the sorrow he felt at that moment. How can a young child learn about death for the first time in this way, particularly that it happened to the person he loved the most?

Emotional trauma can reveal underlying mental health conditions. We often live with our latent disorders and complexities, but when we experience trauma, we lose our mental balance and become overwhelmed by negative emotions. These emotions not only affect our mental well-being but our physical health as well. It is curious how the brain, with its regulated electrical charges and the chemical compositions of hormones, can be so easily disrupted by trauma or extremely negative emotions! The brain would possibly create visual or auditory hallucinations in an attempt to fill the dark void that is left after losing a loved one. Or perhaps it is the brain's way to console the person who experienced that loss.

The complex nature of emotional trauma and its mental and physical effects is not fully understood. However, it certainly has a profound impact on us. Whether it be in psychiatric wards, coronary care units, or in our day-to-day lives, the root causes of trauma exist, which were deeper and more intense to comprehend at the time we experienced them, leaving a lasting detrimental effect on us.

Regardless of the physiological or psychological mechanism of emotional trauma response, and even in the simplest incidents of our daily lives, it can be difficult to limit the damage caused by negative emotions. If we realize that these emotions will dominate our thoughts and determine our future, how can we overcome them?

In his book *How to Become a Human*, Dr. Sherif Arafa presents what he calls "The Emotional Control System[1]." It is a model through which he explains three basic steps to overcome a situation that triggers negative emotions in us. The first step is to learn our lesson. Any situation, emotion, person, or trauma affects us because it carries a message that only those who think deeply about it can comprehend.

Looking for a lesson to be learned from negative experiences is like being armed against negative emotions. This does not mean that negative emotions will disappear completely. Yet, focusing on understanding the lesson can indicate hope of positive emotions that may reduce the burden of negativity and help create a balance between rationality and emotions. Studies have shown that in contrast to experiencing sequential negative emotions solely, having simultaneous conflicting emotions, such as the feeling of loss as a negative emotion and recalling happy

---

(1) Arafa,Sherif.HowtoBecomeaHuman.Cairo,AlDarAl Masriah Al Lubnaniah, 2014,Pp.317.

memories as a positive emotion, can help reinforce the process of overcoming unpleasant emotions and increase an individual's ability to deal with distress[1].

If we could not identify the veiled lesson, we would move on to **the second step**, which is to determine the desired emotion. Currently, we are feeling the weight of loss, and it is becoming too much to bear. So, we need to ask ourselves what we want to feel and experience instead. This leads us to **step three**, which is the Processing System.

In this step, we need to go through three important stages. Reception is the first stage. It involves focusing on receiving only the important information (from the outside world) that is relevant to the desired emotion we set up previously. The second stage is translating the information obtained in the previous stage. Here, it is essential to remember that our interaction with specific information or emotions depends on our own choices.

(1) Araniecka, Anna, Ewa Trzebinska, Aneta Dowgiert, and Agata Wytykowska. "Mixed Emotions and Coping: The Benefits of Secondary Emotions." PLoS One. 2014 Aug 1;9(8):e103940. doi: 10.1371/journal.pone.0103940. PMID: 25084461; PMCID: PMC4118988.

The last stage is action. It means acting like a happy person by practicing meditation and relaxation, distracting our mind by thinking about something else, listening to music, doing some activities, and the like, or resorting to positive catharsis through exercise, for example.

Will this seven-year-old practicing his hobby every day help alleviate the impact of trauma? Could putting our emotions under a scheduled, rigorous system help us control them, minimizing their impact on us, or would they inevitably govern us?

Dear Nurse Um Sakina,

A nurse in the health center

I would like to express my gratitude for the effort and time you put into assisting every mother who comes to vaccinate her child. I greatly appreciate the way you approach each mother with care and attention, starting by inquiring if she was a new mother and then offering advice with the tenderness of a mother and the knowledge of a nurse.

You possess the qualities of a compassionate mother as well as a knowledgeable nurse, which makes your assistance even more valuable. Once again, thank you for your dedication to your work.

I am Feeling Stressed!

When we observe fish in the water, camels in the desert, bears in the ice, and blossoms in spring, they may seem stationary with unchanging habits and constant search for sustenance. They found their safety in adaptation long ago. When threatened, even by a minor occurrence that disturbs their physical and psychological convenience, they do not retain their placidity until that threat is eliminated.

Analogously, we humans strive to find our comfort zone where we can align with internal and external factors. However, any change, be it negative or positive, can disrupt our comfort zone and throw us into a state of chaos where we feel lost, as if sailing in the wind until we find a safe place to land.

This adaptation has three dimensions: physical, psychological, and social, which are susceptible to stress. Any bodily injury, distracting work pressure, or even a boundary-crossing relationship can all lead to an imbalanced adaptation.

Inside operating theatres, I always cared to examine patients' reactions before administering anesthesia. I believe that there is nothing more tense than that moment. I recall a foreign worker in her thirties who entered the cold, strongly illuminated room, and she was all eyes before her gaze finally rested on the LED OT light it lit up. When I approached her, I saw signs of tension on her innocent face. Since she neither spoke Arabic nor English, I could not help her the way I usually did by telling other patients to read verses from the Qur'an to calm their anxious hearts. So, I simply held her hand and smiled at her. She seemed to be a bit relieved as she rushed to declare that she no longer wanted to go through the operation and would rather leave the operating theatre on the spot. I tried to ease her tension with simple phrases, hoping she would understand me, but she refused to calm down until she inhaled the anesthetics and fell asleep. Another patient expressed her nervousness by asking me to stay with her, even if she was unconscious, while the third decided to spend the time praying to God Almighty.

We all experience countless moments of stress in our lives, whether it be in our daily routine when facing major shifts in our personal or professional lives or encountering any internal or external changes. To help reduce and avoid stress, I discovered a tool developed by the Heart Math Institute(1). It looks like an earpiece, except that it is a sensor attached to the lower part of the ear, and instead of amplifying sounds, it records the electrical signals produced when your heart beats through an app. This app is designed by the Institute and is called "Internal Balance." It helps determine if an individual is under stress by analyzing heart rate variability.

The tool and app, then, provide breathing exercises and other information to help manage stress. It is a useful tool for identifying areas of stress and improving the individual's flexibility in dealing with panic attacks.

I have tested this application on myself, some colleagues, and

(1) Since 1991, the HeartMath Institute has developed reliable, scientifically validated tools that help people reduce and avoid stress while experiencing increased peace, satisfaction, and self-security with the help of professional medical staff.

family members, and found that most of their stress was related to daily life. Common causes included financial issues, future plans, social roles, family dynamics[1], and work relationships among other causes. After each session, I would ask if they were practicing any stress-reducing mechanisms, but I rarely received satisfactory answers. Some people associate relaxation with certain social classes and believe that it is not effective for them. Others, on the other hand, unknowingly practice effective coping mechanisms recommended by several psychiatrists to avoid the harmful physical and psychological consequences of chronic cumulative stress.

Coping mechanisms are important in protecting individuals from harm, whether it be physical, psychological, or social. They also enhance individuals' ability to face difficult situations through self-renewal and relieving chronic stress to avoid future impacts. Here are some of these mechanisms[2]:

(1) Out of curiosity and not to conduct scientific research or the like.

(2) Townsend, Mary C. Psychiatric Mental Health Nursing: Concepts of Care in Evidence-Based Practice. Philadelphia, F.A. Davis Company, 2014, Pp. 8-9.

1. Awareness: It is the cornerstone upon which the rest of the mechanisms are built. Without awareness of the problem that causes stress, it is impossible to develop potential solutions and put them into action. By recognizing stressors, individuals can choose to ignore them, avoid them, or accept them.

2. Relaxation: each person has a way of relaxation that does not necessarily work with others. Some people find relaxation in engaging in physical activities, such as sports, while others prefer swimming or even doing house chores. Others use deep breathing exercises or other techniques.

3. Meditation: It is recommended to practice meditation for 20 minutes once or twice a day. Several studies demonstrate that meditation can help reduce high blood pressure permanently, among other stress-related symptoms. Meditating often requires a specific posture and breathing pattern, closing the eyes, attaining calmness and mindfulness, and focusing on a single object, word, sound, or phrase that has a positive meaning for the individual.

4. Seeking external support: Sometimes, simply talking about your problems with a supportive person can greatly reduce

tension. If you cannot find someone to talk to, you can write down your emotions in a journal or diary.

5. Problem-solving skills: By examining the unpleasant situation objectively, you can effectively address the problem that needs to be solved. You can use problem-solving models and make decisions that are found in books and websites.

6. Pet keeping: Recent studies suggest that people who care for pets have a greater ability to deal with stress. This may be due to the compassion and unconditional love that comes from taking care of another living being.

7. Music: Another recent study shows that music helps individuals feel soothed and happy, change their mood, and reduce stress. For Muslims, listening to or reading the Holy Qur'an can even have a deeper impact.

Of course, I'm not saying that you should do exercises in the middle of surgery or bring a little puppy to face a big problem.

Surgery and problems in life are all sources of stress and anxiety. Thus, practicing coping mechanisms has scientifically and practically proven to be vitally important in helping us take control of our actions rather than giving in to the negative impacts of stress and tension. When we get used to these strategies, we can achieve a better quality of life. Instead of expecting others to solve our problems, we can help ourselves by utilizing these mechanisms.

Dear Dr. Abdul Qader,

An Anesthesiologist in the Division of General Surgery

I appreciate your commitment to shaking hands with the patient before every operation. The incident when you removed your medical gloves and a surgical mask to show your face and shake hands with the patient on the operating table left a lasting impression on me.

Knowledge is not Enough

As we journey through life, we encounter many challenges. While we easily overcome some of them, others remain inescapable and may force us to accept our weaknesses as temporary comfort zones compatible with the current stage.

I have experienced moments of weakness like everyone, and I have seen them on the faces of many others. Here in the CPR emergency room, a twenty-seven-year-old man came to the hospital on foot after finishing his work hours at school because of severe pain he felt in his chest. As soon as he entered the hospital, he fell to the ground and was quickly carried and resuscitated. He was revived, praise be to God, but his condition was unstable. Despite the return of his blood circulation to its course, his vital signs were still abnormal, and he had shortness of breath.

Throughout the ordeal, we stood by his side, holding his

shoulders as he struggled to breathe. Even with our best efforts, most of the medical staff felt helpless. There was nothing more we could do to help him if all the medications and devices did not help. We could only rely on the power of God, which is greater than anything. However, every time one of his relatives visited and saw that he was still alive, they felt relieved and happy. The doctor would try to keep them hopeful until they revealed that they worked in the health sector. He would then frankly describe his medical condition, using medical terminology to explain everything in detail.

I believed that what the doctor did could be harsh yet beneficial to the patient and effective in consoling his family. However, this perception drastically changed when the grandmother of one of my close friends was admitted to the intensive care unit. My friend chose to return to this ward, as if she were still an intern, to stay by her grandmother's side until she passed away. She described how she felt at the time, and although I was grieved by her loss, her words were shocking to me. She was the gloomiest of spirits when she was telling us how the doctor's consolation turned into declaring painful facts. After he learned that she studied a medical specialty, she said with eyes full of tears: "I hated nursing and that I studied nursing. I wished I was ignorant of all the terminology he used!"

Despite her passion for this specialty, studying it was the reason why she had to understand the reality of her grandmother's condition. So, she loathed it at times when she was more in need of consolation than knowledge of physiological facts and medical measures.

I certainly do not mean to accuse them of intentionally causing harm; perhaps some believe it is out of transparency and integrity. Others may believe that it promotes rationality and refutes sentiments that weaken the individual! So, are sentiments really in opposition to rationality? Is being sentimental synonymous with weakness? Is an emotional person frail and a rational person strong?

Daniel Goleman, a psychologist and an award-winning author for his Emotional Intelligence, has a different perspective on this matter:

"A view of human nature that ignores the power of emotions

is sadly shortsighted. The very name Homo sapiens, the thinking species, is misleading in light of the new appreciation and vision of the place of emotions in our lives that science now offers. As we all know from experience, when it comes to shaping our decisions and our actions, feeling counts every bit as much—and often more—than thought. We have gone too far in emphasizing the value and import of the purely rational—of what IQ measures—in human life. For better or worse, intelligence can come to nothing when the emotions hold sway. And that is the problem: academic intelligence offers virtually no preparation for the turmoil—or opportunity—life's vicissitudes bring. Yet even though a high IQ is no guarantee of prosperity, prestige, or happiness in life, our schools and our culture fixate on academic abilities, ignoring emotional intelligence, a set of traits—some might call it character—that also matters immensely for our personal destiny[(1)]."

According to Howard Gardner, a Harvard psychologist and the author of Multiple Intelligence theory, "People with IQs of

(1) Goleman, Daniel. Emotional Intelligence. 10th ed., Bantam Books, 2007, Pp. 24.

160 end up working for people with IQs of 100." He believes that while the former group has a high percentage of intelligence, they lack the interpersonal intelligence the latter group has. In today's world, as Gardener suggests, there is nothing of greater importance than interpersonal intelligence[1].

Emotional intelligence is not limited to relationships, understanding the nature of emotions, or knowing how to love. It also extends to five essential areas:

- Intrapersonal intelligence means being able to fully understand oneself and effectively regulate and identify one's emotions, and it is the cornerstone of emotional intelligence.
- Managing emotions: This involves being able to regulate emotions so that they do not spiral out of control. One should be able to calm themselves down in the face of anxiety and respond appropriately to the situation.
- Self-motivation: It is the peak of managing our emotions. It is about our internal drive to achieve a goal by delaying satisfaction and suppressing emotional reactions.

---

(1) Gardner, Howard, Frames of Mind: The Theory of Multiple Intelligences. New York, Basic Books, 1983, Pp. 66.

- Interpersonal intelligence: the ability to understand and interact effectively with others. It involves effective verbal and nonverbal communication. It is especially crucial for those seeking leadership roles.

- Empathy: It is an essential human skill that enables one to read and identify the emotions of others. It is the essence of emotional intelligence.

Throughout history, there have been many different interpretations of empathy. According to the theory of Edward Bradford Titchener, an American psychologist, "Empathy stemmed from a sort of physical imitation of the distress of another, which then evokes the same feelings in oneself(1)." This, according to him, sets a distinction between empathy and sympathy, which "can be felt for the general plight of another with no sharing whatever of what that other person is feeling(2)." On the other hand, Martin L. Hoffman, an American psychologist

---

(1) Goleman, Daniel. Emotional Intelligence. 10th ed., Bantam Books, 2007, Pp. 121.

(2) Goleman, Daniel. Emotional Intelligence. 10th ed., Bantam Books, 2007, Pp. 122.

who is primarily focused on the development of empathy and its relationship with moral development, insists that "empathy must be embedded in moral principles." When people feel the sadness of others, it motivates them to act through moral principles, such as providing support, whether moral or material.

How admirable this sounds! It is greatly relevant to our work as a medical staff, which is focused on providing support and alleviating the sufferings of others. But do we ignore this fact? Why are we unsympathetic at times?

Hoffman conducted an experiment at Princeton Theological Seminary to answer the question: Why don't we take advantage of our many opportunities to help others?

He asked students to give a sermon and split them into two groups. The first group gave a sermon about helping a stranger in need, while the second group gave randomly selected sermons. They were then asked to move to another building to deliver their speeches. On the way, they encountered people who were suffering and wailing. So, did they stop to help them?

Unfortunately, they did not! Despite that, they meditated and preached about helping those in need; they did not help because either they were in haste or their minds were preoccupied with something else.

However, we can avoid such simple reasons by being mindful of our surroundings and offering even the smallest forms of help, such as empathy, to those who deserve it. A nurse may believe that administering medication is the only way to help a patient, while a doctor may insist on a particular operation to alleviate suffering. Yet, simpler opportunities to help may arise, and it is essential to remember that knowing how to help is insufficient if it lacks empathy. Empathizing with others will lead the way for our moral principles to do their work.

Dear Nurse Fatima,

A nurse in the inpatient surgical unit

I am thankful for your appreciation of the simplest things we do. After helping her one day, I will never forget how she took the time to go to the nearby store to buy us sweets as a thank-you gift.

Pizza Every Saturday!

Amidst the monotony of work at the health center, the attending doctor and I took a moment to chat. We talked about general concerns, such as the nursing specialty and the future opportunities it offers. The doctor was very emphatic when she advised me not to miss the academic opportunity. “Do not do as I did. I got tired and dropped the anchor,” she said. At first, I thought she meant her age, although she seemed young to me! Maybe she was talking about her long years of experience. I tried to tell her that she still had a lot to give and there were opportunities that she could take advantage of. She looked away as if contemplating and revealed: “I do not mean aging… I have multiple sclerosis[(1)].”

---

(1) Multiple sclerosis (MS) is a potentially disabling disease of the central nervous system that disrupts communication between the brain and the body. This leads to a number of symptoms, including organic or cognitive-mental symptoms which sometimes appear in the form of psychological disorders.

I have always read about Multiple sclerosis and mentioned it before as a serious disease similar to a frightening nightmare. Thus, I never expected to meet someone successful in their career while dealing with the effects of this terrible disease, let alone a doctor. Despite the challenges of examining patients and diagnosing diseases, the doctor also had to tackle the distressing and depressing symptoms of multiple sclerosis, especially since these symptoms can vary greatly in severity from one person to another. While some people may experience only fatigue and numbness, others may become paralyzed and suffer a loss of vision.

She started experiencing weakness in her lower limbs, which made her motionless for days. She described feeling pain in her feet. Eventually, the pain spread throughout her body, causing fatigue and lethargy from time to time. As a doctor, she believed that medication would be the key to a successful treatment. Unfortunately, it was not, as each capsule of medicine represented a compressed dosage of mental exhaustion, even if it helped her to push the weight of fatigue and pain. She even had suicidal thoughts to end her suffering.

She found a way to prevent her suicidal thoughts from overcoming her mind by being immersed in the concerns of life. She did a lot of research to figure out an effective treatment for her condition. Until she finally realized that the treatment was within her reach! It is, in fact, within everyone's reach, which is to modify some of their eating habits. She specifically refrained from sugar, chicken, cheese, and milk, only to be dazzled with the results. Fatigue and bodily pain disappeared, and the weakness of her feet became less frequent, so she decided to abandon medications and settle for this new approach that provided her with satisfactory results.

She was able to confirm the effectiveness of her approach when the pain returned a few weeks later. She felt disappointed and thought that her dietary plan was failing her and that she had no choice but to take medication. However, she tried to go over her daily routine and meals to see if there was something that she could avoid. She discovered that her family had recently adopted a new habit: eating pizza every Saturday. Unfortunately, the pizza was always covered with a thick layer of cheese, which she realized might be the reason for the return of pain in her feet.

Cheese was one of the foods she had been avoiding, so she had to resist the temptation to eat the pizza. When she stopped eating it, she noticed that her physical and psychological health improved, and she no longer felt fatigue and pain.

Many of us struggle to avoid harmful habits while striving to acquire good ones. However, the habit loop can be both strong and unpredictable. As Charles Duhigg stated in his book The Power of Habit[(1)], “Habits can be as much a curse as a benefit.” Habits are a curse because the brain’s dependence on automatic routines can be dangerous, even if the habit is harmful and life-threatening. Conversely, habits can be beneficial because they often save us valuable time and effort. Without habit loops, our brains would shut down, overwhelmed by the minutiae of daily life, and we would have to expend immense mental effort on basic daily activities. Having work stored automatically in our minds (habits) frees up our time and energy for more important and fulfilling tasks.

---

(1) Duhigg, Charles. The Power of Habit. Random House Books, 2013.

Establishing new habits can lead to positive results, just as breaking existing habits can be beneficial, like when the doctor started taking her tea with no sugar. But how do we form habits, and how can we train our minds to adopt new ones?

The habit loop has three main components. Firstly, there is the cue that triggers habitual behavior and prompts the brain to switch to automatic mode to determine which habit to use. Secondly, there is the routine, which refers to the habit. It may be physical, mental, or emotional. Lastly, there is the reward, which helps the brain associate this specific loop with a reward to remember in the future: "Habits can be as much a curse as a benefit." Habits are a curse because the brain's dependence on automatic routines can be dangerous, even if the habit is harmful and life-threatening. Conversely, habits can be beneficial because they often save us valuable time and effort. Without habit loops, our brains would shut down, overwhelmed by the minutiae of daily life, and we would have to expend immense mental effort on basic daily activities. Having work stored automatically in our minds (habits) frees up our time and energy for more important and fulfilling tasks.

Establishing new habits can lead to positive results, just as breaking existing habits can be beneficial, like when the doctor started taking her tea with no sugar. But how do we form habits, and how can we train our minds to adopt new ones?

The habit loop has three main components. Firstly, there is the cue that triggers habitual behavior and prompts the brain to switch to automatic mode to determine which habit to use. Secondly, there is the routine, which refers to the habit. It may be physical, mental, or emotional. Lastly, there is the reward, which helps the brain associate this specific loop with a reward to remember in the future [(1)].

For instance, if you want to establish the habit of eating healthy every day, you need to start by reinforcing the cue that triggers this habit. This could be a signal that reminds you of the importance of healthy eating, such as keeping healthy ingredients in your kitchen, attaching a note to display the benefits of nutritious foods, or placing the weighing scale nearby to regularly check on your weight.

---

(1) Duhigg, Charles. The Power of Habit. Random House Books, 2013, Pp. 28.

Once the cue is triggered, you can prompt your brain to adopt habitual behaviors automatically. For example, this could happen by preparing a healthy recipe every time you see the healthy ingredients (the cue) or planning an upcoming meal every time you read nutritional tips.

Finally, when it comes to the habit of preparing healthy meals, the reward refers to how the behavior makes you feel satisfied. Then, you need to repeat this loop to reinforce routines and help the brain keep habits firmly in place without any effort.

Speaking of healthy eating, it is a habit that many people strive to establish, but why is it that despite the majority's attempts to eat healthy, eating junk remains pleasurable, and the brain refuses to give up its cravings? The answer lies in the power of reward! Although all habit loops have the three components of cue, routine, and reward, their strength varies according to desire. The stronger the desire for a reward, the more difficult the habit is to break. Desire is one of the principal constituents that nurture and strengthen habit loops. In other words, if you have a greater desire to enjoy the taste of sugar in your tea than to feel satisfied after drinking a sugar-free tea cup, then the habit of drinking sweetened tea will be stronger than the habit of drinking sugar-free tea. Similarly, if the doctor desires the taste of pizza more than the refreshing feeling of having a salad recipe, she will not hesitate to eat pizza every Saturday.

Habits are just as important as the big decisions we make about our health and life in general. In fact, habits are an advanced stage of decision-making. John Dryden believes, “We first make our habits, and then our habits make us.”

I had the pleasure of meeting a doctor who, despite going through painful details, now sits before me with her lovely, gentle personality. She constantly moves around her small clinic and spares no effort to attend to each patient. All this is possible because she established a new habit that brought her back to life.

Let’s take a moment to reflect on the quality of the habit loops in our lives and strive to establish new habits that can help us renew our lives.

Dear Aziz,

The Anesthesia Technician in the operating room

Thank you because attending to your patients was driven more by fatherly love than performance of duty. Your dedication eases patients' anxiety before going into surgery.

Our Unique Strengths

The Egyptian poet, Ahmed Shawqi wrote:

"How did you find your long residency in your last resting place?

I am filled with bitter sorrow and unceasing anguish since you left.

My grief for your death changed me and made your flesh decay.

Yet, your love remains in my heart, unchanged.

Thus, I shall keep my vows to you until the day we gather again,

And you have to uphold them until Judgment Day."

Despite being exposed to serious medical cases and witnessing uncontrollable sobbing, seeing the patients' families next to them and trying to do anything to get them back to life was the most painful moment for me. It is as if I am laying my rational thinking aside and resorting solely to my heart to handle the situation. So many times, I have seen noses redden and eyes sunken to see a loved one with whom they shared the details of the day and night while lying on a bed of a neutral color. A loved one who is incapable of reacting with them or even looking at them and whose communication with the world takes place only through the tubes that surround him.

A seventy-three-year-old patient, whose file contained many acronyms and abbreviations that represented endless complications, suffered from diabetes, high blood pressure, and kidney failure. A heart attack caused her to be in a drug-induced coma that delivered her to a deep and permanent state of unconsciousness. We were used to seeing the patient's husband inside the division, moving hastily between one doctor and another to inquire about her condition. His constant movement stopped only when he settled by her side. He was willing to give up everything for her sake. He brought a chair with him, placed it next to her head, and spent about an hour sitting quietly, just contemplating her. He sat still, and I would say that he was careful not to let her be out of his sight even for a second, as if he wanted to capture as many images of her inside his mind as possible. He then decided to take this hand out of his lap and place it on her left shoulder. I thought that he meant to say, "It's okay. I am not lying by your side, but I am with you, heart and soul, even if my body flounders around among the crowds!

He looked closely at her face and observed her features for a while, then he stretched out his hand and placed it on her forehead, trying to feel her temperature. He immediately rushed to ask: "Why is her temperature so low? You have to measure it at once!" His panic did not cease even after we had done as he asked. It never bothered me because I knew what it meant if the temperature dropped and what it could lead to. He sat beside her for a little while, and his eyes spoke volumes as he gazed at her with fear. Perhaps she, herself, had words that were left unsaid. Maybe she wanted to ask him after he adjusted her veil: "Do you still find me beautiful?" She might have wished to hold onto his hands when he was leaving. Perhaps she wanted to say, "Stay a bit longer! Only you can keep warm in this dreary place. The coldness of death is inevitable."

Another fifty-year-old patient was lying in the blackness of a coma due to increased intracranial pressure from bleeding in the brain. It started with an unbearable throbbing headache, and she vomited as soon as she was in the emergency room. Her two daughters stood outside the room. After several attempts to convince the doctor to allow them in, he finally agreed. The doctor explained the mother's condition to them. One of the daughters surreptitiously took a bottle of water out of her purse, to which, I believe, she had read verses from the Holy Quran. Using her palm, she started wiping her mother's face with that water time and again. The other daughter continued to recite the Qur'an while holding her mother's hand. They were trying to eliminate the darkness of this place spiritually and keep their mother company through the remembrance of God.

Last but by no means least, there was a brain-dead patient who continued to receive people committed to visiting her amid work hours, as the few visiting hours scheduled by the hospital administrator were no longer sufficient for them. We were often used to seeing the son of this patient and his reporting of all of his mother's involuntary movements to the attending doctor, hoping that the doctor would, even falsely, tell him that his mother was just comatose and could wake up with time or treatment to get out of that coffin-like bed. However, the doctor always confirmed that his mother's movements were either impulsive reflexes or the effects of medications and did not indicate that her brain had restored its damaged functions.

I once stopped to watch that son stroking his mother's head and insistently repeating: "Mother, wake up!" Three words he used to plead with his mother, which revealed the pain he felt in his heart and his frustration, followed by his hurrying departure, and everything inside him was crying except his eyes! Day after day, the patient's visitors grew in number, and their sadness increased. Eight family members were with her on her last day. They were so heartbroken that they almost drowned in their own tears. However, I was surprised to learn that the family had signed a do-not-resuscitate order if her heart stopped because they did not want their mother to suffer even from chest compressions.

Although these situations were heart-wrenching and grievous, I felt a strong bond with these people. It urged me to think about those who tragically died alone without being surrounded by their loved ones.

All these spiritual emotions, empathy, compassion, and concern, are points of strength in the human personality, as described by the American psychologist Martin Seligman. He studied all major religions and philosophical traditions and found that all human cultures shared the same six virtues. Some scientists defined them as knowledge of the basic things in life. Seligman classified them into six categories:

1- The virtue of wisdom and knowledge include creativity, curiosity, love of learning, open-mindedness, and perspective and wisdom.

2- The virtue of courage encompasses various traits such as bravery, Persistence, integrity, and vitality.

3- The virtue of humanity is accompanied by strengths like love, kindness, and social intelligence.

4- The virtue of justice comprises team spirit, fairness, and leadership.

5- The virtue of temperance includes forgiveness and mercy, humility and modesty, Prudence, and self-regulation and self-control.

6- The virtue of transcendence is accompanied by strengths such as appreciation of beauty and excellence, gratitude, hope, humor and playfulness, and spirituality or sense of purpose.

When we exhibit courage or compassion, we are using the strengths that can only be found inside us. Moreover, some writers argue that interdependence, cohesion, empathy, and harmony are also personal strengths. However, I find that one of the most profound descriptions of human strength is being able to do our best in the most challenging situations(1). So, can we say, despite our broken hearts and frailties, that we are still capable of using our human strengths?

---

(1) C.R. Snyder, Shane J. Lopez, and Jennifer Teramoto Pedrotti, Positive Psychology the Scientific and Practical Explorations of Human Strengths. Sage Publications, 2011.

Dear Dr. Maryam,

A physician in the Emergency Department,

I appreciate your spontaneity and modesty towards patients. Despite your busy schedule in the emergency room, you always remember to ask the patients to pray for God to grant you success in your endeavors.

The Cornerstone of Life

As you read these words, someone in the world is reciting love poems; another is perhaps dancing to love melodies; and someone else may be shedding tears because of love. Love is a formidable force that can revitalize our lives as much as it can destroy them!

For centuries, human beings have been on a quest to find love. It is an inexplicable feeling that cannot be seen or measured. People have often resorted to literature and mythology to find an explanation for what they feel. I, too, was once part of this world. One of the first books I owned was a collection of historical love stories I often lent to friends.

I recall trying to write a story that was inspired by this book. My Arabic teacher nominated me to participate in a writing contest at school. She asked me if I had written any literary pieces before. I was embarrassed to say yes and perhaps feared that the teacher's reaction would be harsh. And I was right! You can now imagine a middle school child with a round, innocent face, flowing with kindness, saying in her low voice: "Yes, I wrote a love story!"

As soon as I uttered these words, all I could see was her eyes out on stalks as she screamed, "Love!" I tried to lessen her shock as I rushed to say: "It is about innocent love! Love is not amoral!"

Well, perhaps I was unconsciously defending myself when I said these sentences. However, now, after ten years, my ideas about love have evolved, and I no longer feel that it is an ambiguous, mystifying feeling as I write about it. After spending most of my time in hospital rooms, I discerned steadfast love day-to-day that I could pick up glimmers of love breaking through the doors of these rooms despite the tragic stories.

The first of these rooms was the delivery room! Delivery rooms are mostly known to be painful and horrific places where one can hear countless cries of pain by mothers. Yet, it is equally a place flowing with tenderness and amiability with numerous cries by newborns! When I first entered this ward, I headed to the delivery room. It was medium-sized, with no wall openings from which light or air could penetrate. Five beds were placed inside, and next to each bed was a Doppler apparatus that registered both fetal movements and fetal heart rate, and the ultrasound transducer was placed on the mother's abdomen.

I headed to one of the mothers who was suffering silently despite the varying inconsistent contractions visible on her screen. I approached to greet her and, after praying for her, decided to stay with her for a while. She was a first-time mother. It was evident that increased tension appeared in her eyes as she explored the place and examined the screen of the device. The contractions intensified, and it was time to give birth. She pushed with a lot of pain till she could no longer proceed despite our motivating words. Only when the midwife notified her that the fetus was in danger did she display extraordinary strength to protect her fetus. It is miraculous how pain can inspire so much strength!

After everything she went through, starting from the creation of the fertilized egg in her uterus until the moment in which she experienced unmatched pain, her newborn finally came out healthy. She waited for his crying to ensure that the lungs were working properly, then cried tears of joy as she stretched out her hands, longing to take him in her arms.

I have always wondered how a mother can live the experience of pregnancy time and time again after going through unbearable pains. I then read a quote that goes: "When the midwife finds that a pregnant woman is not in pain during labor; she knows that her delivery is not happening soon. A new life is associated with pain. Just as clay needs fire to solidify, love is incomplete without pain!" Therefore, I realized that I was witnessing the birth of a special kind of everlasting love.

The second room was the operating theatre. As I was passing by one of its windows, I saw an intern doctor repeatedly going back and forth in the room with heavy footsteps. At first, I thought that he was worried about a practical test or probably had made a serious mistake during an operation! Then, when the anesthesiologist came out and patted him on the shoulders to comfort him, I learned that his mother had to undergo a minor surgery (one-day surgery). Although he is a doctor and knows the procedures of the operation, he was restless and worried about his mother.

The last room I remember was the emergency room of the mental health department. I particularly recall the incident when an expatriate man admitted his brother there. He was aware that his brother would lose his job for being a mental health patient, but he was only interested in his therapy regardless of the consequences.

In the next room, a sedated patient was lying in one of the beds. At the side of the bed sat his brother, speechless and motionless, just contemplating his brother, with whom he shared his childhood and life, helpless and bedridden.

But what is love? It is an interesting question that has equally intrigued many scientists and curious individuals. In an article written in 1986 titled "A Triangular Theory of Love,[(1)]" psychologist Robert Sternberg suggests a "triangular" concept of love that comprises three key components: intimacy, which

---

(1) Sternberg, R. J. (1986) "A Triangular Theory of Love." Psychological Review, 93, 119-135.

involves the desire for closeness, connectedness, and bondedness; passion, which involves romance and the physical relationship; and commitment, which is the intention for a long-lasting relationship.

According to Sternberg, consummate love comprises all three components and is the total form of love. Moreover, the presence of one component or a combination of two components creates other kinds of love experiences, such as romantic love, which bonds people emotionally through intimacy and physical passion but lacks commitment. On the other hand, infatuation is characterized by physical passion without liking or commitment, while empty love is characterized by commitment without passion or intimacy.

Other psychologists adopted different definitions of love. According to Freud, love and work are the cornerstones of our humanness." This means that, as human beings, we need to love and feel loved. This idea is also supported by an ancient Indian philosophy that promotes three sides of human life: self-sustenance, self-actualization, and love.

Neuroscientists have also studied love and its effects on the brain. They have discovered, through radiography, that certain areas of the brain are activated during the experience of love. For example, when women fall in love, the activity in the centers responsible for rational thinking, fear, and anxiety decreases. Conversely, the activity in the areas responsible for intuition and memoryincreases.[(1)]

Whereas scientists define love using neurological terminology, poets define it in emotional vocabulary, philosophers use the sublime language of philosophy to define it; mothers, meanwhile, uniquely express their love through the language of their children; and for me, love is conveyed through acts of compassion and humanism.

So, what is your own definition of love?

Love is within us. The biology of love originates in the primitive parts of the brain. It is the core of our humanity. We

(1) Insel, T.R. and Fernald, R.D. (2004) "How the Brain Processes Social Information: Searching for the Social Brain." Annual Review of Neuroscience, 27, 697-722.

have the power to express it in our own unique way. Thus, we are free to live love the way we want rather than limit it to the feelings shared between a man and a woman. Regardless of the love you choose, always remember to ask yourself, “Is this how love should be?»

Dear Operation Theatre Technician Ahmed

Technician in the Division of General Surgery

I would like to express my gratitude for your kindness towards children. I am particularly impressed by the way you initiate interactive conversations with them often by asking the question: “Are you a Hilal supporter or a Nassr supporter[1]?”

(1) Saudi football teams.

The Eyes Look, but the Brain Sees

Amidst the monotony of repetition in my days, there comes a unique day that breaks the endless cycle of daily routine. Days, as such, bear lessons to be learned in life, and missing this valuable opportunity would be a waste of time and effort. These thoughts were going through my mind as I planned to visit a special place and meet new people of different mindsets and attitudes. Our diversity adds colors to our lives, making them brighter and more vivid.

But what about you? Do you live in a grey existence? Or do you add colors to your world?

Colors are a way to visually distinguish between objects and realize their beauty. However, some of us have lost the ability to perceive this distinction. They chose to discover beauty through other means and excelled in capturing it in the most overlooked places.

It was time to visit our friends at Al-Noor Institute for the Visually Handicapped, and we prepared simple informative content on healthcare to present. However, I was worried about this visit and feared that I would offend the visually impaired by treating them with pity. Nevertheless, as we got to know them closely, I had the chance to recognize their potential and creativity. My perspective shifted, and I realized that my pity was unwarranted altogether. Rather, I felt pity for myself, not for them.

We divided them into small groups to present the healthcare content we had prepared while moving between these groups. We also interacted with the members of each group, holding their hands through the practical application to ensure the information was delivered effectively. It was now their turn to showcase their skills and the potentiality of their institute. Initially, I had a limited idea of the institute's scope, believing it only taught blind women how to use Braille devices[1]. However, I discovered that

(1) It is an electro-mechanical device for displaying braille characters, usually utilizing round-tipped pins raised through holes in a flat surface. Visually impaired computer users can use it to read text output.

these devices were merely tools they carried around, the way we carried pens with us and that they utilized them to learn the same curriculum taught at any other school. Indeed, I was amazed by the well-equipped laboratories that catered to their specific needs.

Their honorable teacher handed us a thick book that seemed to be empty! As I had a closer look, I noticed the raised dots, which they could read with their fingers as their course books. I tried to touch these dots, but my hand could not feel them, and perhaps my brain refused to help me! The book contained a map of the world drawn with dots as well. There was an animal anatomical model, as well as leaflets with illustrations of human body parts printed on one side and a measuring tape with a compass on the other side. The collection of materials in their laboratory helped students draw a picture of the outside world in their imagination, not through their eyes, but through their little fingers. Perhaps their picture of the world was more vivid and beautiful and allowed them to live freely, as this approach enhanced the students' non-visual abilities and heightened their other senses.

Helen Keller was an American writer, lecturer, and activist who experienced hearing and vision loss when she was twelve months old. She believed that “”character cannot be developed in ease and quiet. Only through experience of trial and suffering can the soul be strengthened, ambition inspired, and success achieved.””

We all need to go through experiences, such as my experience with a tool I picked at the Al-Noor Institute. It was a wooden board with six gray raised dots that represented the twenty-eight letters of the Arabic language in Braille. I tried to solve its mystery, and then I found out that some of these dots could be hidden while others were left behind to form each letter separately. Many students tried to help me read one of the letters. After much effort, I finally managed to read the letter alef, which was represented by a single dot.

I left the institute with a lot of ideas and recalled one of my favorite books, The Brain That Changes Itself, by Canadian psychotherapist Norman Doidge. The book describes how the brain, far from being fixed, has endless adaptability and remarkable powers to change its structure and compensate for challenging neurological conditions. Despite the controversy which surrounded the main idea of the book, it is definitely worth reading. Doidge discusses the work of neuroscientist Paul Bach-y-Rita, who proposed the concept of sensory neuroplasticity. He suggests that if one of the senses is damaged, sometimes another sense can compensate for it through a process called "sensory substitution[(1)]."

Bach-y-Rita's experiments gave great hope to the blind, as he states that "we don't see with our eyes, we see with our brain." He explains that the eyes are just the receptors of light energy, whereas the brain interprets the signals of the senses to determine what we are looking at.

One of Bach-y-Rita's most famous inventions was the "tactile vision substitution system," the most revolutionary invention in 1969 in sensory neuroplasticity. It was a chair similar to a dentist's chair, connected to a camera that enables the user to recognize the object coming towards it. The camera would then send electrical signals about the image to plates resting against

(1) Doidge, Norman. The Brain That Changes Itself. Penguin Books, 2008, Pp. 27.

the blind user's back. The signals sent to the brain from the skin via touch were being processed in the visual cortex because of the way the patients interpreted the information.

The tactile vision device was a groundbreaking invention in the field of neuroplasticity, and it brought about a significant improvement in the lives of the blind. Doidge describes the device: "A large old dentist's chair with a vibrating back, a tangle of wires, and bulky computers. The whole contraption, made of cast-away parts combined with 1960s electronics, weighed four hundred pounds (180 kg)[(1)].»

Later, the machine was transformed into an electronic chip that could be conveniently placed on your tongue instead of carrying a hefty weight equivalent to the weight of a sumo wrestler. This revolutionary chip is now known as the "brain port" and has become a boon for many visually impaired individuals, helping them to carry out various activities with ease.

These thoughts brought me to one of the TED talk videos

---

(1) Doidge, Norman. The Brain That Changes Itself. Penguin Books, 2008, Pp. 24.

titled "Can We Create Senses for Humans?" by neuroscientist David Eagleman. He was inspired by Paul Bach-y-Rita's idea, but instead of helping the blind, he adapted it to help the deaf. He did this by connecting a voice recorder to an electric chip attached to a vest that the deaf person can wear anywhere. The chip translates external sounds into electronic signals that stimulate the wearer, with each letter or word having a different stimulation until a sentence with meaning is formed. The vest has had remarkable results, as demonstrated by a video of one of Eagleman's trainees who, on just his fifth day of training, could write down the words he heard seconds after hearing them. Eagleman concluded: "We have been very encouraged by our results with sensory substitution, but what we've been thinking a lot about is sensory addition. How could we use a technology like this to add a completely new kind of sense, to expand the human umwelt?"

It's both unfortunate and impressive that the inventions in this field have greatly advanced in such a manner, while I still struggle to run my fingers over the lines that a blind student at the Al-Noor Institute wrote to me using the Braille device. I try to read it with my eyes closed at times and take a close look at the raised dots at other times. At last, I discovered what she had written: "Thank you for today, Noura Al-Subaie. That was really informative."

I truly hope that one day, one of these inventions will be used at the institute. And when that day comes, I will write back to you: "Thank you for opening new windows through which I can take a fresh look at the world."

Dear Dr. Youssef,

A Neurologist

I truly appreciate the hard work that has led you to become a successful neurologist. I have often observed doctors discussing and arguing about various cases, and it is impressive to see when they consult with you, how quickly you would give an accurate diagnosis.

Will He Choose to Stop His Heart?

Have you ever found yourself overwhelmed with your plans? You become in a state where you are sleep-deprived because of the anxiety you feel about one of your goals. Even the most spacious places seem narrow when you feel lost in your thoughts. We are often indecisive regarding the decision we are compelled to make but have terrible, and sometimes justified, fear of its consequences.

I still remember that patient who was brought by his brother to the CPR in the emergency department one afternoon. The young man was suffering from heart palpitations accompanied by dyspnea and fever, which deprived him of sleeping, eating, and even sitting still. Unfortunately, this was not the first time. He had a heart disease and had been attending medical appointments. His vital signs showed that his heart rate exceeded 200 beats per minute, while a normal resting heart rate for adults ranges from

60 to 100 beats per minute. His heart condition was confirmed by the electrocardiogram and electrocardiographic imaging carried out by the medical staff. The doctor immediately described a triple dose of beta-blocker medication to manage abnormal heart rhythms and started other medical procedures, but to no avail! The doctors' medical terminology was getting sharper and more complex! And their hand gestures revealed that they were arguing about something! They finally made their decision to use low-energy DC shock (direct current cardioversion) to treat him. However, it is there is even a slight chance of cardiac arrest. How is that for a consequence?

A simple one! Isn't it? It simply means that the muscle responsible for pumping life into the body will stop for a moment... Or, possibly forever? On the other hand, this direct shock that should regulate heartbeats may help to restore a normal heart rhythm. This did not come as a surprise to his brother, who had thoroughly studied his condition and the possible procedures. However, he was tongue-tied, and almost everyone in the room realized the fear in his eyes as they gazed at his brother and then at the rest. At last, he decided to break the awkward silence to give his agreement to the doctors' decision.

It is common to experience lots of different emotions when making an important decision, like confusion, worry, and sometimes even fear of the possibility of what might happen. It is also common to hesitate in fear of making the wrong decision until we become paralyzed and unable to make any decision at all. So, what are the barriers to decision-making?

According to Dr. Sherif Shehata, who has written extensively on the topic of decision-making, there are eight obstacles: self-deception by exaggerating or neglecting facts, external factors and the opinions of others, previous ideologies, low self-esteem, indolence, blame-shifting, spiritual apathy and feeling disconnected from God, and finally, psychological issues.

Sometimes, our emotions or latent desires can lead us to deceive ourselves by exaggerating or neglecting facts when making decisions. Therefore, we become blind to certain details, whether voluntarily or involuntarily, which could change the course of that decision, perhaps due to fear of the consequences of acknowledging these details. To make the best decision, it is essential to determine our primary objective and examine all the details with a fair and impartial eye. By doing so, we can expect that an effective decision will made.

External factors and opinions of others play a key role in the decision-making process. We all have a person who has influenced us, such as a family member, friends, media, and education. An influential person can have a great impact on our thoughts and decisions. Yet, there is no harm in turning to someone for advice. (No disappointment shall be the lot of one who seeks Allah's guidance, nor does one regret if he seeks advice[1]), but without allowing others to make our decisions for us.

Moreover, previous ideologies, which are the set of beliefs and ideas that shape our understanding of the world around us, can greatly influence our decision-making. However, it is important to know that using the same mechanisms and ideas every time will not lead to different results.

Lacking self-confidence and being trapped in indolence could also profoundly impact our lives by causing us to turn

(1) Hadith by prophet Mohammed, mentioned in Nahj-al Fasahah, compiled by Abu l-Qasim Payanda.

down opportunities and lead us to inaction. We may miss out on many chances, fearing to expose our points of weakness to others. Additionally, blame-shifting might be a mechanism used to retain our status or avoid shame. We tend to shift the blame for our bad decisions to external factors, whether it be people, life incidents, or timing. We may have high self-esteem, but indolence often holds us back from achieving our goals.

It is important to realize that tomorrow or next week may not be the best time to start our pending tasks. We may use the excuse that the task will take up too much of our time as a reason not to start it. However, if we take the first step, we will often find that it takes less time than we thought.

All the reasons mentioned above are trivial compared to our deep faith in God Almighty if we believe He only chooses what is good for His servants. Even if God's preferences seem to be not in our best interest, he only forbids us to do certain things for a reason. If we are unable to do something, it is because of some wisdom that we are unaware of. Thus, it is important to establish a mechanism that can help you regain faith in God. For instance, I always try to do something three times in different ways, and when I am unable to do it, I stop and forget about it, believing that God has a better plan for me.

In case you are wondering about the heart patient, after receiving DC shocks, he woke up with a healthy heart and regular heartbeat.

Dear Nurse Fatima,

Nurse in the Internal Medicine Inpatient Ward

I wanted to express my gratitude for your dedication to prioritizing the patients' needs over your own convenience. I still remember how wet wipes became a popular choice among nurses for cleaning patients to save time and effort. However, you chose to use soap and water instead, explaining that "it is a cleaner and safer option for the patients."

Will You Show Me a Ray of Hope?

Have you ever felt a sudden loss of direction in life? It is as if you have been stripped of all your principles and self-complexities. You feel caught between the past and the present moment or trapped in a labyrinth where you are desperately going in circles. You have no clear path to follow, but you are dragged to a situation you have never encountered before. I could read all these feelings in the eyes of a patient during my first with her at the mental health hospital.

As soon as we entered the inpatient ward, we encountered this patient. She walked with slow, heavy steps as if she was hoping that life would surprise her and stop what was happening in her present to bring a new order to her life. This behavior made us apprehensive at first, especially since it was our first encounter with a mental patient. Soon after, our caution turned into deprecation when she seemed disinterested in everyone around her and barely acknowledged our presence, unlike the other patients. I thought she was schizophrenic because she seemed aimless, fatigued and depressed. However, when I asked one of the patients about her. I learned that she was not suffering from any psychological disorder. Rather, she was in a mental hospital due to a legal situation that remained unknown to us to this very moment.

We moved to the living room with the patients after each group of us was assigned to be responsible for one patient. We started introducing ourselves to bridge the gap between the staff and the patient, which is the core of therapeutic communication as a key mental health practice. This approach is based on choosing a certain type of questions to get the desired answers or detect signs of disorder through the way they talk and move from one conversation to the other. I worked with two of my friends with a schizophrenic patient. I could not join their conversation, though, as my mind was occupied with the patient, who later turned out to not be a patient. I was thinking: Is it possible that a mental health hospital should be used as a penal institution when dozens of people try their best to convey the substantive objective of psychotherapy and demystify misconceptions about it? On the other hand, I felt very sorry for her; how must she feel now in a place where she does not belong and with people with whom she is estranged?

As I got lost in my thoughts, I noticed that a woman had taken a seat next to me despite the plenty of empty chairs in the room. I turned to see it was the inpatient that occupied my thinking. Trying not to seem too curious, I smiled and asked how she was doing. Her behavior revealed that she was nervous and struggling to shake off a disturbing nightmare. Her legs would not cease shaking, and worry lines appeared on her forehead, distracting the attention from the dark circles under her eyes. She tried to start a conversation by asking me about our training. I was glad she asked and answered as thoroughly as possible, trying to show her that I was interested in talking to her. I then asked her why she was in the inpatient ward, but her sweet smile turned into a shy and disappointed one. She refused to reveal the reason. I hastened to tell her that we could talk about something else to avoid any unwanted embarrassment. However, she only smiled briefly before continuing her mysterious quest in the department's corridors.

I spent nearly an hour and a half talking with patients while watching her. I regretted not choosing a better time to ask my question. Later on, snacks were given out, which consisted of pieces of cake and juice. All the patients started eating immediately except the inpatient, who came back to sit beside me. She took a few moments to look at her cake, split it in half and smiled while handing me the other half. I sensed that perhaps she wanted to tell me: "I trusted you… I will give you cake, and you will show me hope!" Maybe she wanted to prove to me that she was a good person and hoped I could help her get out of the place. I kept thinking of the possible words she had never uttered until my day with her came to an end, and it was the first and last day I saw her.

After a whole year had passed, we had to return to the mental health hospital with new roles and different plans. As soon as we entered the inpatient ward, I looked among the faces in an attempt to find that patient. I felt happiness and fear at the same time when I did not find her. Is she home now? Or was it moved to another, more mysterious place? The supervisor in charge smiled bitterly when I asked her about the patient. She told me that she was discharged, but after she had turned into a mental patient during her last days in the hospital. She started behaving like them, relieving herself on her clothes, unconsciously stripping naked, and unfortunately, she attempted suicide twice.

I felt a shiver running through my body as I stared at her, not believing what she was saying. She seemed normal to me; she was nice and well-behaved. So, what happened? Is it the weight of despair? Did depression find its way to her? All I got for an answer was that she was only impacted by the patients around her.

The nurses who attributed what happened to the patient to the influence of mental patients around her may have been referring to the theory of psychologist Gabriel De Tarde on social learning or the laws of imitation, as he termed it. This theory was further elaborated by the famous psychologist Albert Bandura, who defined social learning as an individual's acquisition of new responses or behavioral patterns within a social situation or framework. Bandura's theory suggests that learning inevitably takes place in a dynamic and reciprocal interaction of the cognitive context, environment, and behavior.

Moreover, Bandura states that human behavior, with its personal and environmental determinants, forms an interlocking system of mutual and interacting influences.

One of the key aspects of this theory, which particularly interests me, is "observational learning." Bandura believes that "from observing others, individuals form an idea of how new behaviors are performed, and this coded information, consciously or unconsciously, serves as a guide for action[1]. According to him, observing others involves learning and adopting new behaviors because learning occurs through observation, imitation, and modeling. As individuals communicate and get into contact with each other, they imitate each other because they observe the actions of others and copy them. This leads to learning new behaviors from one another.

It's important to realize that not all of our behaviors result from conscious decisions. Sometimes, imitation and social learning play a key role in learning new behaviors. Yet, the responsibility to consolidate our cognitive abilities falls upon us

---

(1) Engler, Barbara. Personality Theories: An Introduction. Pennsylvania, Houghton Mifflin, 1985, Pp. 366.

to assess whether a behavior is positive or negative and avoid being mere products of our environment.

Tell me now, dear reader! Do you think that the patient would have done better if I showed her a glimmer of hope in exchange for her cake?

Dear Nurse Maryam,

A Nurse in the Intensive Care Unit

I genuinely admire that you were among the first nurses to emphasize the importance of talking to patients, even if they were unconscious or in a coma. While assisting you with your duties, I can never forget how you used to have long conversations with patients who may not be able to respond.

Emotional Wounds

The rays of the scorching sun reflected on the blue walls of the internal medicine inpatient ward. It is the department where all the medical diagnoses and clinical examinations take place. Each part of it includes ten rooms with two to three beds each. The beds are rarely devoid of patients because internal medicine is a specialty that deals with a broad and extensive number of diseases. Therefore, if an intern were looking for a certain medical condition, they would definitely find it in this ward.

However, some of these medical cases remain vague, with insufficient details to understand what happened and unclear visible signs to explain the patient's condition.

One case is of a fourteen-year-old girl who had attempted suicide by taking a number of her grandmother's blood pressure and diabetes pills because of a fight with her friends. Despite her appalled and innocent gaze, and with all the love her mother showed towards her and the great fear she felt even when we checked her daughter's vital signs, she, unfortunately, tried to take her own life.

There was also another seventeen-year-old girl who was admitted because of seizures, which everyone thought to be epileptic. Nonetheless, after being examined by a neurologist, it turned out that she was having psychogenic nonepileptic seizures. This diagnosis led her father to think of all the incidents that may have caused it, such as sitting alone sometimes and the way the school principal dealt with her provocatively for no apparent reason.

Lastly, a woman over thirty years old was admitted because she was initially diagnosed with multiple sclerosis. The symptoms included pain in the right side of her body and paresthesia associated with headaches that affected her face and blurred her vision as well. These pains were accompanied by exhaustion and fatigue when making the least effort. After completing the medical examination, it turned out that she did not have multiple sclerosis but one of the migraine attacks. Since I, too, suffered from migraine, I asked the doctor about its symptoms and causes, and he told me that the latest research suggested that this disease was associated with sensitive or creative people. (It is no secret, dear reader, that I was happy to hear that, even though I was feeling a terrible headache in the right half of my head at the time.)

It is worth bearing in mind that a wide range of medical conditions can be affected by psychological factors. Therefore, research on this topic was not limited to migraine but also included several diseases caused by psychological stress. Needless to say, psychological stress can dysregulate the human immune system and, consequently, our general health. For instance, a German doctor named Ryke Greed Hamer reviewed the files of his cancer patients and found a correlation between types of cancer and psychological causes. For example, he suggested that constant marital conflicts could lead to breast cancer, and the constant fear of the future and persistent thinking about death could lead to lung cancer.

I then remembered an interesting idea presented in one of the TED talk videos titled "Why We All Need to Practice Emotional

First Aid?" by psychologist Guy Winch. He emphasizes the importance of "emotional hygiene", which is parallel to personal hygiene. Just like we take care to clean a wound in our body to prevent contamination and promote healing, we should also be mindful of cleaning up our psychological wounds. Why do we tend to downplay the significance of emotional pain, such as depression, when we don't do the same for physical injuries? For instance, if you are feeling depressed, people tell you, "Just shake it off; it is all in your head." Can you imagine saying that to somebody with a broken leg: "Oh, just walk it off; it is all in your leg."

By correcting this misconception, we surmount the first stage of emotional hygiene. The next stage is the most challenging one, which is identifying our harmful psychological habits and changing them the way we change our unhealthy physical habits. One of the most dangerous habits is accepting negative thoughts such as failure, rejection, and self-deprecation. Dr. Mary J. Lore, in her book *Managing Thought*, refers to these thoughts as "destructive and diseased thoughts" that make our minds ill, hinder their progress, and cause emotional wounds that are hard to heal. To avoid accepting these thoughts, Lore recommends three rules that help us determine whether our thoughts are good or destructive. This technique can be called "emotion filtering", and it is similar to how we filter water to keep impurities from getting into our bodies. Thus, Lore lists three simple questions to filter our thoughts:

1- Does the idea bring me safety or inspire me?

2- Does the idea cause harm to me or others?

3- Does it help or hinder our progress? (1)

If the answers to the first and third questions are negative and the answer to the second question is positive, the thought you have is, unfortunately, diseased and contaminated. In other words, by not eliminating it, you are exposing yourself to psychological injury sooner or later. This, in turn, plays a key role in developing many physical diseases such as heart disease and others.

---

(1) Lore, Mary J. Managing Thought: How Do Your Thoughts Rule Your World? Ferne Press, 2008, Pp. 57.

By applying Lore's rule to all the thoughts that represent psychological influences in our lives, we can identify good thoughts that will strengthen our emotional immunity and psychological state - God willing. Hence, the average life expectancy will increase, just like it had risen within a few decades by 50% a hundred years ago when people started paying attention to personal hygiene and physical cleansing. Imagine how much higher it could go if we also pay attention to our psychological hygiene.

Dear friends,

Nurses in different wards,

I am thankful for having you as my best companions along this path of knowledge and work.

The Function of the Ego

Have you ever tried to search for cake or candy bars inside a hospital? If you have not been to a health fair, then you have missed out.

Not a single academic program goes without awareness exhibitions or participation in health forums within health centers and hospitals. As part of a nurse's responsibility for health education, these activities were essential to us.

Today, we are holding an awareness forum in the hospital's lobby, which was lit by the sun. We have come equipped with information and learning rules to give our presentations. The turnout has been good so far, and we have been able to help many people. However, after a few minutes, the number of participants decreased.

I noticed someone from afar who seemed to be looking for

something. I did not know what it was until he approached us. Instead of asking us about the exhibition and the information it presents, he asked: "Isn't there any cake?" I will not say that I was shocked, but I felt great discontent; people's desire for delicious foods is not something new or strange at all, but associating (some) health forums and awareness activities with serving unhealthy foods is strange.

Do not be surprised, dear reader, when you attend a lecture on diabetes to find the types of cakes and sweets. So, do we mean to challenge a diabetic patient to a test of will?

Do not be surprised either to see all kinds of candy wrapped in pink ribbons served when attending a forum on breast cancer, as if we are ignoring recent research that directly links sugar to cancer!

I certainly do not mean to underrate the forums or the lecturers but rather disapprove of the prevalent contradictory interrelation between healthcare awareness and unhealthy habits. A couple of my friends attempted to design a simplified education program targeting diabetic and high-blood pressure patients at a health center. They decided to give out small bags to keep medicines instead of the usual sweets and thought it would be more helpful because of the large number of tablets used by diabetic and blood pressure patients. I liked the idea very much, and I expected that many would welcome it, but the reactions were disappointing. Most people found the idea strange and made fun of it, as they expected sweets to be served or pies at least. This experience made me realize how difficult it can be to change unhealthy habits.

The organizers of healthcare programs were probably aware of the contradiction but could not help it. This paradox is just one of many that can create a lot of conflict and confusion in our lives. It permeates every aspect of our being and affects our choices and attitudes.

Sigmund Freud discovered this contradiction in the human psyche. Freud's personality theory saw the psyche structured into three parts: the ego, the id, and the superego(1). The id represents our instinctual drives, which respond directly and

---

(1) Freud, Sigmund. A General Introduction to Psychoanalysis. Wordsworth Editions, 2012.

immediately to basic urges, needs, and desires. The id operates on the pleasure principle that every unconscious wishful impulse should be satisfied immediately, regardless of the consequences. It is primitive, illogical, irrational, fantasy-oriented, and has no comprehension of objective reality. It is mostly expressed as aggression and violence.

The ego's primary purpose is to preserve life. It prevents danger and employs anxiety to control instinctual drives. It operates according to reality principle to satisfy less dangerous primitive desires, often compromising or postponing satisfaction to avoid negative consequences of society. The ego engages in secondary process thinking, which is rational, realistic, and orientated toward problem-solving.

The superego restricts satisfaction, guiding behavior towards moral righteousness. It incorporates the values and morals of society, which are learned during one's childhood. The external authority of parents or educators is transformed into an internal psychological authority, inducing guilt when standards are not met. The superego is the voice of conscience (doing what is right) and the source of self-criticism.

Moreover, the ego is responsible for the minutiae function of mediating between the instinctual desires of the id and the moral constraints of the superego, and any failure to create balance between them can result in disorders.

This confirms that these three authorities are the source of the contradictions that we often experience, but without which balance cannot be achieved. Have you ever been torn between eating a candy bar (id) and maintaining your health (ego)? Or, have you ever wanted to satisfy an instinctive desire (id) but feared to distort your self-image (superego)?

As is the case in health forums, we may experience this contradiction! On the one hand, we caution patients about sugar consumption, but on the other hand, we choose to serve sweets to welcome guests. Therefore, to create balance, we must consider all three structures of the psyche to make the right decision that satisfies our ego. Let's say it is acceptable to serve delicious dishes to guests as long as they are made of healthy ingredients.

Dear reader,

A tiny letter of gratitude to all of you who took the time to obtain and read this book. I genuinely appreciate your time and commitment.

Afterward

As I was about to complete writing this book, I received a message on a social media platform from someone asking me about nursing. She had been accepted into nursing school despite not preferring it. I explained to her the advantages and disadvantages of nursing. Our conversation ended with her feeling satisfied and grateful for being accepted into this specialty. A few days later, she messaged me again with another question: "Is it possible to transfer from nursing to medicine school?" This made me wonder if my story would be lived by others in the future.

Bibliography

Arafa, Sherif. *How to Become a Human*. Cairo, Al Dar Al Masriah Al Lubnaniah, 2014.

Araniecka, Anna, Ewa Trzebinska, Aneta Dowgiert, and Agata Wytykowska. "Mixed Emotions and Coping: The Benefits of Secondary Emotions." PLoS One. 2014 Aug 1;9(8):e103940. doi: 10.1371/journal.pone.0103940. PMID: 25084461; PMCID: PMC4118988.

Benson, Nigel. *The Psychology Book: Big Ideas Explained*. DK Publishing, London, 2011.

Benson, Nigel, Joannah Ginsburg, and Voula Grand. *The Psychology Book: Big Ideas Simply Explained*. New York City, DK; First Edition, 2012.

Covey, Stephen R, *The Seven Habits of Highly Effective People:*

Restoring the Character Ethic. New York, Simon and Schuster, 1989.

Claros, Edith, Kimberly Foisy, and Teresa Deam *Nursing History and Theory*. Jones and Bartlett, 2013.

Doidge, Norman. *The Brain That Changes Itself*. Penguin Books, 2008, Pp. 27.

[edited by] Donna D. Ignatavicius, M. Linda Workman, Mary A. Mishler. *Medical-Surgical Nursing across the Health Care Continuum*, 2013.

Duhigg, Charles. *The Power of Habit*. Random House Books, 2013.

Engler, Barbara. *Personality Theories: An Introduction*. Pennsylvania, Houghton Mifflin, 1985.

Freud, Sigmund. *A General Introduction to Psychoanalysis*. Wordsworth Editions, 2012.

Gardner, Howard, *Frames of Mind: The Theory of Multiple Intelligences*. New York, Basic Books, 1983, Pp. 66.

Gerbner, G., Gross, L., Jackson-Beeck, M., Jeffries-Fox, S., & Signorielli, N. (1978). "Cultural indicators: Violence profile," no. 9. Journal of Communication, 28, 176–207.

Goleman, Daniel. *Emotional Intelligence*. 10th ed., Bantam Books, 2007, Pp. 24.

Insel, T.R. and Fernald, R.D. (2004) "How the Brain Processes Social Information: Searching for the Social Brain." Annual Review of Neuroscience, 27, 697-722.

Kubler-Ross, Elisabeth, and David Kessler. *On Grief and Grieving*. New York, Scribner, 2005, PP. 20-35.

Lore, Mary J. *Managing Thought: How Do Your Thoughts Rule Your World?* Ferne Press, 2008, Pp. 57.

Nikolajsen L, Jensen TS. "Phantom Limb Pain," British Journal of Anaesthesia. 2001; 87: 107-116. Ketz AK.

Okasha, Ahmed. *Physiological Psychology*. Cairo, Dar Elmaref, 1986, Pp. 67.

Quilliam, Susan. *What Makes People Tick?: The Ultimate Guide to Personality Types*. Element, 2003.

Shehata, Sherif. *Decision Making*. Giza, Dar Al Raya, 2016, Pp.19.

Sternberg, R. J. (1986) "A Triangular Theory of Love." Psychological Review, 93, 119-135.

Townsend, Mary C. *Psychiatric Mental Health Nursing: Concepts of Care in Evidence-Based Practice*. Philadelphia, F.A. Davis Company, 2014, Pp. 8-9.

www.ingramcontent.com/pod-product-compliance
Lightning Source LLC
Chambersburg PA
CBHW031344230926
51848CB00002B/380
* 9 7 8 6 1 4 4 2 9 5 4 3 4 *